KINESIOLOGY

Maggie la Tourelle is a holistic health therapist, teacher and writer. She started teaching Touch for Health, basic kinesiology, in 1984 and since then has gained wide experience in all the main branches of kinesiology. She has also trained in many other branches of the healing arts including Neuro-Linguistic Programming (NLP).

Anthea Courtenay is a freelance writer, journalist and translator. She specializes in the field of natural medicine and healing, and has written for a number of magazines and publishers.

IN THE SAME SERIES:

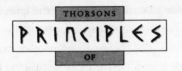

THORSONS
PRINCIPLES
OF

KINESIOLOGY
TOUCH FOR HEALTH

MAGGIE LA TOURELLE WITH ANTHEA COURTENAY

Thorsons
An Imprint of HarperCollinsPublishers

The publishers would like to thank Jillie Collings for her suggestion for the title of this series, *Principles of ...*

Thorsons
An Imprint of HarperCollins*Publishers*
77–85 Fulham Palace Road,
Hammersmith, London W6 8JB
1160 Battery Street,
San Francisco, California 94111–1213

Originally published as *Thorsons
Introductory Guide to Kinesiology* 1992
Published by Thorsons 1997

3 5 7 9 10 8 6 4 2

A catalogue record for this book
is available from the British Library

ISBN 0 7225 3454 X

Printed and bound in Great Britain by
Caledonian International Book Manufacturing Ltd, Glasgow

CONTENTS

ACKNOWLEDGEMENTS

I would like to acknowledge the inspirational work of Dr George Goodheart, the creator of Applied Kinesiology. I would also like, on behalf of students and lay practitioners, to acknowledge with deepest thanks the vision and generosity of Dr John Thie and Dr Sheldon Deal. My thanks also to Dr Bruce Dewe for his interest in and support of this book, and to Elizabeth Andrews for kindly lending her expertise in reading the manuscript. Finally, I am grateful to all the teachers and practitioners who have so kindly contributed essential information to this book.

Maggie la Tourelle
London
November 1996

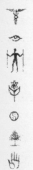

FOREWORD TO THE FIRST EDITION

*P*rinciples *of Kinesiology* provides both the general public and health professionals with an understanding of this new approach to health promotion which has been developing over the last twenty-nine years.

Modern scientific medicine is outstanding in caring for severe injuries and works very well in the diagnosis of tumours, cancers and infectious diseases. However, it has developed and specialized to such a degree that people suffering from functional rather than infectious or pathological problems often need to see several different specialists, and may still end up without a satisfactory outcome.

I often hear it stated, and I agree, that in the United States modern medicine is the fastest-growing failing business in the world. Its costs are increasing at three times the rate of inflation while at the same time there are more cases than ever before of infant mortality, arthritis, musculoskeletal problems, headaches, and other conditions which cause loss of productivity as well as loss of happiness. At the same time, with increased longevity more and more people are suffering from chronic conditions which the scientific medical approach does not seem to address adequately.

Another approach had to be developed. To fill this need the new field of Kinesiology has come into being along with other complementary methods of health promotion and disease prevention. As a participant in this changing paradigm I have seen Kinesiology help millions of people in all parts of the world, from emerging nations in Africa and South America to all the industrialized nations and the former Communist block. I know of no other complementary health promotion modality that has grown so fast and spread so widely.

The Touch for Health synthesis which this book describes may contain just what you, the reader, needs to help yourself, your family and friends. This approach sees the human being as a co-operative part of the whole, and assumes an intelligent design with a purpose for everything in the universe. It allows for, and even forces, new ways of asking questions, and different ways of working than are currently available in the scientific medical approach.

One most important process that is now emerging is the changing attitude of the medical establishment. These highly intelligent professionals also recognize the need for a change in the paradigm within which they have been operating. As professionals in the scientific medical field become aware of this new complementary paradigm, they are also recognizing its value; some are learning to practise it themselves, and others are referring patients to practitioners and to classes at which lay people can learn to help themselves.

This book may change your life for the better. Reading it will give you a complete background, while the case histories may include descriptions of problems relevant to yourself or your family or friends. Kinesiology and Touch for Health offer a very safe approach to health care, and the possibility of learning to help yourself to greater health and well-being.

My hope is that more and more people around the world will be able to empower themselves through these methods, so that the human race can continue to develop and fulfill its purpose more effectively. I urge you to join us.

John F. Thie, D.C.
Bloomington, California, U.S.A.
March 28, 1993

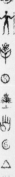

INTRODUCTION

Kinesiology is one of the fastest growing and most interesting developments in modern natural health care. It is a system of health care that uses muscle testing as a diagnostic tool, and treats the whole person using a combination of gentle, safe techniques. It spans the full spectrum of health and healing, from its physical application in chiropractic, osteopathy and sports medicine to the less tangible areas of psychotherapy and healing. With its remarkable range of applications, linking the physical aspects of health to the emotional and spiritual, Kinesiology is becoming a vital ingredient of health care in the 1990s, both as a therapy in its own right and as a complement to orthodox medicine and other therapies.

Since its inception in 1964 by the American chiropractor Dr George Goodheart, Kinesiology has developed and expanded into an extraordinarily wide variety of fields. Today it is practised throughout the world by doctors, dentists, chiropractors, osteopaths, naturopaths, physiotherapists, nutritionists, counsellors and many other natural health care practitioners, as well as businesspeople, educationalists and laypersons. Since 1973 Touch For Health, a system of Kinesiology developed specifically for non-professionals, has been experienced by well over two million people in at least 42 countries.

With its use of manual muscle testing, combined with other diagnostic techniques, Kinesiology offers one of the best methods of assessment (some practitioners would argue *the* best) available in modern health care. Unlike many other therapies, which claim to be holistic but are biased in favour of one particular technique or philosophy, Kinesiology is truly holistic. It encompasses all aspects of the human being – the structural, nutritional and psychological components of health – and provides a means of assessing and correcting imbalances in all three, often interacting, areas. Its combination of muscle testing techniques, holistic approach and effective treatments enables Kinesiology to obtain positive results when other approaches, including orthodox medicine, have failed.

ABOUT THIS BOOK

This is an information book covering the wide scope of Kinesiology; it is not intended to be an instruction manual, although some self-help techniques are included in Chapter 6. It has been written for the general public and for prospective students and health practitioners – of both orthodox and complementary medicine. It is for those who have little or no previous knowledge or experience of Kinesiology, and will also be of interest to those who have experienced one branch of Kinesiology and would like to know more about its wider applications. A list of organizations, training schools and contact people is given in Appendix B.

In countries other than the USA the largest number of practising Kinesiologists are natural health care practitioners who have recognized the potential of Kinesiology but are not qualified to give a medical diagnosis. Kinesiology has also been taken up by a smaller number of medically trained people, including doctors, dentists and physiotherapists. The practice of Kinesiology varies from country to country depending both on historical factors and on current legislation. In the USA, where it originated, it is practised mainly by people who have a licence to diagnose, such as chiropractors, osteopaths, doctors and dentists.

This book aims to give an overview of Kinesiology as it is currently used, including Applied Kinesiology, Touch For Health, and other applications that are taught and practised world-wide. Included are descriptions of the ways in which muscle testing is used and of correction and treatment techniques, together with a discussion of the very wide range of conditions that Kinesiology can correct or improve, from the physical to the emotional, from nutritional deficiencies to learning difficulties, and from full professional care to self-help techniques. This book also includes a range of case histories showing the variety of ways in which people have benefited from Kinesiology in its different forms. These case studies are culled from the personal experiences of Maggie la Tourelle and her colleagues; some minor details and the subjects' names have been changed to protect their confidentiality (and in those cases where 'I' or 'me' is used this refers to Maggie la Tourelle).

Maggie la Tourelle
Anthea Courtenay

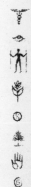

SOME DEFINITIONS

Kinesiology, as will be seen, provides a very direct way for the practitioner to communicate with the patient or client, and vice versa, through the body. At the same time, as is true of other forms of conventional and alternative medicine, Kinesiology has acquired a specific verbal language of its own, and it may help the reader at this point for some of this terminology to be explained.

WHAT IS KINESIOLOGY?

The word 'kinesiology' comes from the Greek word *kinesis*, which means 'motion'. In the medical sciences it is the name given to the study of muscles and the movement of the body. 'Applied Kinesiology' was the name given by its inventor, Dr George Goodheart, to the system of applying muscle testing diagnostically and therapeutically to different aspects of health care. Today the name Applied Kinesiology (AK) refers only to the parent system, as taught by the International College of Applied Kinesiology (ICAK). As a number of different branches have evolved, the term Kinesiology has come to be accepted (outside the medical profession) as a general term for all these systems.

Kinesiology could be defined as follows: Kinesiology is a system of natural health care which combines manual muscle testing with the principles of Traditional Chinese Medicine (TCM), energy balancing and other healing modalities. It is truly holistic, working with the inter-relationship between body structure, chemistry, the mind and emotions, and energy systems. Kinesiology assessment uses muscle testing to let the body reveal precisely the location and/or nature of its imbalances, and dictate its preference for treatment. It uses a range of gentle yet powerful corrections and treatments, specific to Kinesiology, which bring about instant change and balance. It can be applied in any field, and draws on and integrates other therapies.

MUSCLE TESTING

We shall be describing muscle testing in some detail, but it is important to understand from the start that in Kinesiology, muscles are tested *not for their strength* as practised in physiotherapy, but to assess the quality of the muscle response.

ENERGY

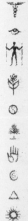

In Kinesiology, as in many forms of natural medicine today, the words 'energy', 'energetic' and 'energetically' have specific meanings rather different from their everyday use. The word 'energy' does not mean 'get up and go' – although increased get up and go often results from a Kinesiology session. In this context energy, also often referred to as 'subtle energy', refers to systems of energy within and around the body.

Subtle energy is synonymous with the *Qi* (pronounced *chi*) of Chinese acupuncture, and with the *prana* of traditional Indian medicine and philosophy; through the ages many other terms have been given to this universal life-force, the harmonious flow of which is vital to the health of mind and body.

Although it has long been disregarded by modern medicine and science, the existence of subtle energy is coming to be much more widely accepted. This is partly due to the Western culture's acceptance of acupuncture, and partly due to technological developments such as Kirlian photography, which produces prints of the subtle energy field and shows variations that reflect variations in the health and energy of the subject.

Today the terms 'Energy Medicine' and 'Vibrational Medicine' are being increasingly applied (by doctors as well as natural therapists) to a whole group of natural healing systems, which include acupuncture and Kinesiology. An excellent and very thorough book has been written on the subject by the American MD, Dr Richard Gerber: *Vibrational Medicine: New Choices for Healing Ourselves* (Santa Fe, NM: Bear & Co., 1988).

Such subtle energy has always been seen and felt by sensitive people such as healers, and acupuncturists are trained to read to flow of *qi* through twelve specific pulses on the wrists. These are connected with a series of energy pathways called *meridians*, each relating to specific bodily organs, glands or systems.

In Kinesiology a further connection has been made between meridians and specific muscles, with which they are 'energetically' connected. Kinesiology uses manual muscle testing to assess the subject's energy, and then applies a range of techniques to promote the healthy flow of energy throughout the body.

BALANCE AND IMBALANCE

The ancient philosophy of Chinese medicine states that health comes from being in balance and harmony with all things, balance being a perfect state in which no aspect is either deficient

After a pre-professional training at the University of Detroit, Dr Goodheart graduated in 1939 from the National College of Chiropractic which, in his own words, produces 'physicians who use chiropractic methods'. In fact the International College of Applied Kinesiology (ICAK) only accepts students with medical or scientific qualifications.

THE CHIROPRACTIC BACKGROUND

Applied Kinesiology (AK) has its roots in chiropractic. Chiropractic, which means 'done by hand', is a method of manual manipulation of the spine and joints invented by a gifted (if somewhat eccentric) American, Daniel Palmer, in the late nineteenth century. Chiropractic is more than a manipulative technique: it is based on the concept that the nerves are responsible for all body function and therefore interference with the nervous system interferes with healthy functioning. Treating the spine affects the whole person, since the spine encloses the spinal cord and the central nervous system, from which nerves issue to all parts of the body.

Chiropractors are not only concerned with the spine and joints, however; they are also concerned with muscles, since it is the muscles of the body that hold the spine and other bones in position. Weak or over-tight muscles cause deviation in posture and the skeletal system, and can be responsible for problems to recur time and time again after manipulation. It was the underlying need for correct muscle balance that led to the interest in testing for and correcting muscle imbalance and the creation of Applied Kinesiology.

Chiropractic is based on the premise that health comes from within, through the innate intelligence of the body. According to Daniel Palmer, this innate intelligence is connected to the

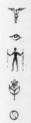

universal intelligence that runs the world; thus the nervous system provides our link to Universal Intelligence.

Today, chiropractic is the most widely recognized alternative therapy world-wide, and is particularly widespread in the USA, where for many people the chiropractor has replaced the family doctor as primary health care giver. In other countries chiropractic has recently been gaining wider recognition; in 1990 the results were published of a clinical research trial conducted by the British Medical Research Council in conjunction with the British Chiropractic Association, showing that chiropractic manipulation is a more effective and longer-lasting treatment of low back pain than is conventional hospital out-patient treatment.[2]

Dr Goodheart was the son of a chiropractor who also practised homoeopathy, allopathic (conventional) medicine, osteopathy and naturopathy, and he was influenced by his father's eclectic approach. In 1964, when he discovered Applied Kinesiology, he was already highly respected as a leader in his field, and was giving regular seminars to his professional colleagues on new chiropractic techniques.

THE FIRST DISCOVERY: EXPERIMENTS WITH MUSCLE TESTING

Dr Goodheart made his discovery, as he put it, 'by sheer serendipity'. He was treating a young man who complained that he couldn't get a job involving manual work; he always failed his physicals because his shoulder blade kept 'popping out'. Examining the muscle that pushed the shoulder blade forward, Dr Goodheart was surprised to find that it was not atrophied from disuse, as he had expected. He also found some painful nodulations (tiny bumps) at the point where the

[2] *British Medical Journal*, 2 June 1990, vol. 300, pp. 1431–1437.

muscle was attached to the rib cage. When he pressed on these they seemed to disappear, and when he massaged them deeply the muscle itself became stronger.

This interesting finding led him to further experiments in testing muscles, using standard methods. Dr Goodheart found that whenever a muscle became weak, the corresponding muscle on the opposite side of the body tended to tighten, 'adding insult to injury'; however, when the weakness was corrected, the tightness or spasm was relieved. This was quite a revolutionary finding: it had always been assumed that muscle spasm came first and caused the weakness on the opposite side. On the contrary, according to Dr Goodheart, muscle weakness often appears first; moreover, this weakness could come about for a number of reasons that had hitherto been unrecognized.

In his muscle testing experiments Dr Goodheart next found that some muscles were weak because there was a sluggishness in the lymphatic system (lymph being the organic substance that feeds and cleans body tissues). When the lymphatic system was stimulated by massaging specific reflex points on the body, the relevant muscles would strengthen.

Over time Goodheart tested muscles in relation to other bodily systems. He found that some were weakened through poor circulation, or from a lack of flow in the spinal fluid, from faulty nutrition, or from disturbances in an acupuncture meridian (see The Acupuncture Connection, below). These finding explained why chiropractic corrections did not always 'hold', so that some patients kept coming back for further treatment. More than that: correcting these weakensses by the appropriate means, such as massage, gentle touch or prescribing vitamins, restored harmony to the body on a more permanent basis. In fact, here was an instant and precise method of both assessing the state of a number of bodily systems and restoring any imbalances found during this assessment.

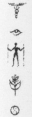

Dr Goodheart began teaching the techniques of Applied Kinesiology to other chiropractors, who adopted them with great enthusiasm.

THE ACUPUNCTURE CONNECTION

One of Dr Goodheart's most important discoveries was that there are connections between muscles, organs, and the acupuncture meridian system.

The acupuncture system was developed by the Chinese sometime between 3,000 and 25 BC. They discovered that disease occurred when the life-force, or *qi* (pronounced chi) is not flowing freely through the body, and they mapped out the *meridians* – the channels or pathways through which this energy flows. Along these meridians lie specific points, called acupuncture points; the flow of *qi* can be balanced by stimulating or sedating these points. Each meridian is linked energetically with an organ, gland or part of the body: a malfunctioning lung, for example, would cause an imbalance in the energy flow of the lung meridian, with which it is linked energetically.

The meridian system is closely connected with the function of the nervous system. Interference with the nervous system caused by illness or stress can cause the loss of signals in the body. Correcting the meridian system assists the nervous system, and thereby the body's communications network, enabling the body to function better.

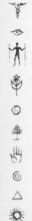

In the early 1970s, after several years of developing and refining Applied Kinesiology (AK), Dr Goodheart was still aware of some unfilled gaps. He began taking a special interest in the medical research of Dr Felix Mann, who had introduced acupuncture to the British medical profession. The connection between meridians, organs and glands was already known; Dr Goodheart's innovation was to find a link between the meridians and particular muscles. He discovered, for example, that a malfunctioning lung would cause an imbalance not only in the lung meridian, but in its related muscle, the deltoid (the muscle on top of the shoulder, which we use to raise our arm).

Dr Goodheart's finding added a whole new dimension to the diagnostic potential of Kinesiology, since a weak muscle could also indicate an imbalance in its related meridian and associated organ and/or gland. The result was the development of Meridian Therapy, which now forms the basis of AK and many branches of Kinesiology.

Dr Goodheart and his colleagues developed a series of muscle tests, based on the muscle-meridian connection. This added a new dimension to the range of corrective treatments already being used, as meridians and acupuncture points could also be used to strengthen weak muscles. Instead of using the traditional acupuncture needles, this strengthening could be achieved through touch. The process is very similar to that for dealing with electrical circuits, in that touching or stimulating certain acupuncture points will make a muscle 'turn on' or 'off', strengthening or weakening it.

To continue with the example of the lung meridian, when there is disease or an imbalance in the lung, the deltoid will show a weakness in a Kinesiology muscle test. Stimulating or balancing the meridian energy, through working either on the meridian or on specific acupuncture points, is one of the treatments applied to restore energy to the lung itself, promoting the healing process. Once treated, muscle strength is also restored, providing a kind of biofeedback which shows that the lung meridian energy is now balanced. This applies to all the meridians and their related organs/glands and muscles.

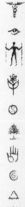

THE TRIAD OF HEALTH

Kinesiology techniques can be used in association with a wide number of therapeutic and other methods, from the physical through the emotional and mental. Used as a complete therapy, it is truly holistic.

Nowadays the word 'holistic' tends to be applied to almost any non-medical therapy, often inaccurately. Some practitioners of natural medicine treat patients by correcting symptoms only, or by focusing on only one aspect of health care – structural, nutritional or emotional, for instance – and ignoring the other aspects. A truly holistic practitioner of either orthodox or natural medicine will take into account not only the patient's physical symptoms but also his or her emotional, chemical and environmental state, all of which contribute to the total picture of health or illness.

Kinesiology, in its complete form, has more right than many therapies to call itself holistic. Kinesiologists look at health from three main viewpoints – the chemical, structural and mental – each of which interacts with the others, and which together represent a whole, in what is referred to as The Triad of Health. For someone to be completely healthy, all three systems need to be functioning well, and in harmony with each other. And, because of their interconnection, the root causes of disease are not always obvious.

For instance, the obvious treatment for back pain might seem to be manipulation (or painkillers); however, if the sufferer also has a poor diet, or is a heavy smoker (which affects muscle tone by destroying Vitamin C), and/or has an unhappy home life, manipulation alone is unlikely to bring about a permanent cure. Similarly, digestive problems may be caused by emotional stress rather than nutritional deficiencies, while anxiety attacks may be traced to a structural or chemical imbalance.

Muscle testing, combined with other Kinesiology techniques, enables the practitioner to find out which of the three systems is out of balance; similarly, Kinesiology corrections and treatment can be applied to all three areas. In fact, restoring the balance can be the key to bringing about profound changes in people's lives.

HEADACHES/MILK ALLERGY

A woman presented herself at a public lecture and demonstration of Kinesiology, suffering from a severe headache. She was a legal worker, unmarried and in her early 30s, and she explained that she suffered regularly from headaches, and was also hyperactive.

A Kinesiology assessment found that she had weak muscles relating to her stomach meridian. Since this was a public demonstration, simple Kinesiology techniques were used to balance the energy in the woman's stomach meridian.

The effects were instantaneous. The woman got up from the massage table announcing that she felt quite different; her headache was gone, and she was clearly much calmer.

She followed this up by going privately for treatment, when further Kinesiology testing revealed a chronic weakness in her stomach muscles. This weakness was traced to a severe allergy to milk. After she cut milk out of her diet, many other aspects of her life improved. Her headaches stopped, she calmed down, and her family commented on the difference in her behaviour.

Nor did the change stop there. Feeling better and thinking more clearly, she studied Kinesiology and decided to train as a naturopath, a discipline in which she could also apply her Kinesiology training. She started a new relationship, left the legal profession, and went to Canada to complete her training in naturopathy.

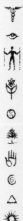

TOUCH FOR HEALTH (TFH) AND APPLIED KINESIOLOGY (AK)

In developing his ideas and research, George Goodheart worked with a core group of chiropractors. One of his closest colleagues was Dr John Thie, DC. Having been involved in the early developments of AK, Dr Thie had a vision of making the amazing, health-enhancing benefits of AK available to everyone. In 1973 his book *Touch For Health* was published. It presented a synthesis of AK techniques in a form that could be understood and safely used by anyone, including people without any medical training or manipulative skills.

Following this, the Touch For Health Foundation was formed; its trustees included George Goodheart, John Thie and Sheldon Deal, DC. The TFH Foundation created a TFH Instructors' training workshop, which trained instructors world-wide. This led to the rapid expansion of Touch For Health, as people from all walks of life all over the world learned and shared the techniques. Since 1973 TFH has been experienced by well over 2 million people in at least 42 countries.

John Thie's aim was for Touch For Health to be available to anyone interested in self-health enhancement, and that it should be shared with family and friends. TFH was never intended as a therapy. However, an increasing number of health professionals took the training, and began incorporating TFH into their practices.

Drs Goodheart, Thie and Deal, all trustees of the TFH Foundation, were also founding members of the International College of Applied Kinesiology (ICAK), founded in 1974. Although George Goodheart supported Touch For Health and its aim of self-help enhancement for laypersons, he became unhappy about the increasing number of non-medically trained health practitioners who were using it.

Thus the TFH Foundation and ICAK grew in different directions. ICAK became the representative body for those wanting a strictly professional organization; it has stringent rules for membership. The TFH Foundation, on the other hand, has continued to represent all those who want to share Touch For Health as widely as possible. Dr John Thie and Dr Sheldon Deal continue to be members of both bodies.

Sheldon Deal, like John Thie, had a vision of making TFH and other Kinesiology techniques available to both medical and non-medical people, who could usefully learn and share them with others. Whereas John Thie created a synthesis of the early developments of AK and called it Touch For Health, Sheldon Deal has created, and continues to create, a synthesis of the ongoing developments of AK, which he calls Advanced Kinesiology and which omits manipulative corrections carried out by chiropractors and osteopaths.

Since the early 1980s, Dr Deal has been teaching Advanced Kinesiology to Touch For Health instructors world-wide. As many TFH instructors are also practising therapists, this has enabled thousands of health professionals to increase their knowledge and skills in Kinesiology, and to pass the benefits of this on to their clients.

Some years ago the orientation of the TFH Foundation changed, and became a research organization. Its teaching role has been taken over by the International Kinesiology College (IKC), which is based in Europe and was originally headed by Dr Bruce Dewe, a medical doctor who is also a member of ICAK. Dr Dewe has expanded the Touch For Health training by developing intermediate and advanced Kinesiology training courses, under the umbrella term Professional Kinesiology Practitioner (PKP) training. These courses also synthesize AK and other techniques, but use different methods from those of Dr Sheldon Deal.

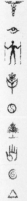

Other branches of Kinesiology have been developed by people whose first Kinesiology training was in TFH; the main ones are described in Chapter 7.

AK TODAY

Applied Kinesiology (AK) remains firmly based in the orthodox field. It is regulated and governed by the International College of Applied Kinesiology (ICAK) in the USA. Because of its chiropractic background, most people training in AK already have a training in manipulative skills, including many chiropractors in the USA and some chiropractors and osteopaths in the UK. Only candidates with four years' full-time training in medicine or the medical sciences, who have a licence to diagnose, may apply for training and membership of ICAK.

AK is defined today as a system of diagnosis and treatment that uses standard muscle testing procedures as an art and science to evaluate body function, and applies a range of approved therapeutic techniques.

AK is an holistic system based on the concept of the Triad of Health. Disturbances of body function, be they physical, mental or chemical, reveal themselves through a change in neuromuscular integrity, and the muscle concerned tests weak under clinical conditions. AK uses the muscle-meridian/organ-gland association as part of its assessment, as well as other specialized Kinesiology assessment procedures. Some of these are described in Chapter 4.

The findings of an AK assessment are always used in conjunction with other standard diagnostic methods, such as taking a medical history, physical examination, laboratory tests and X-rays when appropriate. George Goodheart advocates being a 'diagnostic giant, and then therapy becomes very simple: you know where, when, how and why to do it.'

Correction techniques and treatments used in AK are mainly drawn from chiropractic, osteopathy, acupuncture and other therapeutic disciplines, and unlike TFH and other branches of Kinesiology they include chiropractic and osteopathic manipulation and soft-tissue work for spinal problems. Some of the most common corrections will be described more fully in Chapter 5.

Muscle testing is also used to select effective treatments, and again afterwards, to check that treatment has been effective. A change in the muscle response from weak to strong indicates that the treatment has improved neuro-muscular function.

The initial AK training is 100 hours long and covers a syllabus of ICAK-approved material. All AK research projects presented by teachers of AK are tested in the field for three years before being accepted as approved AK material. Only graduates of ICAK can use the name 'Applied Kinesiology' in relation to their work.[3]

TFH

TFH is a synthesis of early AK material formulated by Dr John Thie especially for people without a medical background or manipulative skills. Its aim is self-health enhancement for everyone through energy balancing. It is not a therapy, and is not used to diagnose or to treat symptoms.

Touch For Health shares many of the basic concepts of AK, in particular the holistic approach embracing the Triad of Health. It is based on energy balancing, using the same muscle-meridian/organ-gland connections as AK, and the same muscle testing technique (though it employs fewer muscle tests). It also shares most of the standard AK corrections, excluding manipulation (see Chapter 5).

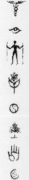

[3] For a more detailed description of AK, contact Applied Kinesiology Seminars UK (see 'International Kinesiology Organizations' in Appendix B).

Touch For Health is the most widely used system of Kinesiology in the world. Training is open to anyone interested in health care. The TFH training was designed for lay people; I have developed a TFH training for practitioners called Foundation Kinesiology Practitioner (FKP). TFH, FKP and similar trainings are recommended as foundation training for people wanting to train in specialized branches, to become professional kinesiologists or to use kinesiology as an adjunct to their own therapy or field. (For details of training organizations see page 175. See also the Summary Chart on page 132 and the content of TFH and FKP workshops and courses in Appendix A.)

The case study that follows is an illustration of the original intention behind Touch For Health. It is good to know that in this day and age, when there are so many budding health professionals, there are still people who love to share TFH without any professional involvement or fees being attached to it.

TFH IN THE FAMILY

A woman in her early fifties watched a demonstration of Touch For Health at an exhibition, and had a short session there, which she enjoyed. Looking round her local holistic bookshop a few days later, she found a copy of John Thie's book *Touch For Health*. Shortly afterwards she attended an evening class I was running on Touch For Health, and when she went home she practised on her family

As a result her sister joined the class, and they had great fun practising together. Then her son joined as well, while another son came to me for individual sessions. Everyone in the family was balanced regularly, including the woman's husband – and the dog! Not only did their health and well-being improve; they all got great pleasure out of sharing this experience, and continue to do so.

HOW KINESIOLOGY CAN HELP

Illness does not arrive suddenly, though it may seem to do so: it is usually the result of a build-up of stress, physical or emotional, leading to imbalances in the body/mind system which ultimately lead to physical symptoms. Regular maintenance with Kinesiology or Touch For Health can prevent this build-up from occurring.

It is not an over-statement to say that practically everyone can benefit from Kinesiology, from the unborn child to the old-age pensioner, from the fit to the infirm and injured – even animals can profit by it.

Whatever the symptoms, Kinesiology balances the body and puts it in the optimum state to heal itself, by removing negative stresses, be they physical, chemical or emotional. Its greatest application is in dealing with everyday complaints for which no permanent cure has been found. About 80 per cent of the problems other than disease that people take their doctors fall into this category. Kinesiology, working as it does from an holistic base, acknowledges the interrelationship of the different bodily systems. The assessment techniques are good at identifying the causes of problems, and can be very useful in pin-pointing the sources of general unwellness and fatigue that are so prevalent today and have no obvious medical cause.

Kinesiology takes the guesswork out of treatment by letting the body reveal precisely where the problem is and exactly what the body needs in order to be healed, so that problems are corrected at source, often permanently. Kinesiology is also ideal for preventive health care, and in its lay version, Touch For Health, can be used by anyone along with his or her family and friends for this purpose.

As well as enhancing the health of the healthy, Kinesiology can help the ill to cope with their illness, in that it enables the whole system to function more harmoniously. People with medical conditions can be helped by Kinesiologists who are trained to treat these more serious conditions; sophisticated Kinesiology techniques can be combined with other diagnostic and therapeutic techniques, enabling people to function as well as possible under the circumstances, and to be supported towards better health.

Kinesiology can even help those who cannot be muscle tested directly, such as small children and babies, and the aged. For this, surrogate testing is used, in which muscle testing is carried out on another person, acting as surrogate. This allows even the injured and unconscious to be helped; it is also useful for animals. Surrogate testing is described in detail in Chapter 4.

Some people who have health problems may need the help of a practitioner who can combine Kinesiology with some other area of specialization. Sometimes different types of treatment may be required at different phases of the healing process; for example, after dealing with structural factors there may be a need to address emotional issues, or vice versa. Sometimes, after an initial assessment or after a period of treatment, a Kinesiologist may refer the client to another Kinesiologist, health practitioner or medical doctor.

WHAT CAN KINESIOLOGY HELP?

Because Kinesiology does not focus on specific symptoms, but tests for and corrects imbalances throughout the whole body/mind system, the list of health problems which it can help or alleviate is endless. Kinesiology corrections encourage the body/mind to heal itself, whatever symptoms are manifesting; indeed, symptoms often disappear without any direct intervention. The following case histories show how Kinesiology can help both the very young and the elderly.

A CHILD WITH POOR EYESIGHT

Jimmy, aged six, was severely short-sighted in his left eye, as a result of a lazy left-eye muscle. When he came to see me he was already attending an eye hospital, where they were very concerned that he might have a serious, permanent problem.

During the assessment I asked him to read a standard eye-chart, with and without his glasses, first with both eyes and then with the right and left eye separately. I recorded how much he could see. The Kinesiology assessment showed an imbalance in the muscles connected with his eyes, and that his eye co-ordination was poor.

I carried out some Kinesiology corrections, consisting of massaging specific acupressure points and reflex areas, and asked him to do a simple eye exercise. At the end of his first half-hour session, when I repeated the same tests with the eye-chart, his sight had already improved so much that he could see as well without his glasses as with them. This meant that his prescription was no longer appropriate.

I advised Jimmy's mother that he should continue with the exercises he had been shown, and that she should take him back to the hospital for a fresh assessment – which she did. She told

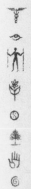

me that the hospital could not understand how such a dramatic improvement could have occurred.

Jimmy has to wear glasses for a slight squint, which is a separate problem. Over a year later the improvement in his eyesight has been maintained, and according to the hospital he has 20–20 vision.

A SENIOR CITIZEN WITH KNEE PAIN

Miss E., aged 75, came to see me about a severe pain in her left knee, which she had had for about a year. An orthopaedic specialist had diagnosed torn ligaments, and she had been treated with physiotherapy and painkillers, followed later by osteopathy, over a period of a year – all with little benefit.

In the assessment I found that a small muscle behind her knee was weak, and was affecting the functioning of the surrounding muscles. After this muscle had been strengthened with standard Kinesiology corrections, the pain disappeared immediately and permanently.

While the specific knee pain has never recurred, Miss E. still has occasional spasmodic stiffness in her knees, and has continued to visit me regularly for maintenance treatments.

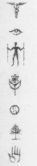

Not all Kinesiology treatments are so instantaneously effective, but such results are certainly not unusual. The list below is intended to give some idea of the scope of Kinesiology.

- Accident trauma
- Addictions
- Allergies
- Anxiety
- Asthma
- Backache
- Bed-wetting in children
- Bladder problems
- Bowel problems
- Breast soreness
- Candida albicans
- Chronic fatigue syndrome (M.E.)
- Constipation

- Co-ordination problems
- Depression
- Diarrhoea
- Difficulty in concentration
- Digestive problems
- Dyslexia
- Ear problems
- Eating disorders
- Eczema
- Emotional upsets
- Exhaustion
- Eye problems
- Fatigue
- Fears
- Flatulence
- Food intolerance
- Frozen shoulder
- Haemorrhoids
- Headaches
- Hiatus hernia
- Hip pain
- Hyperactivity
- ICV (Ileocecal Valve syndrome)
- Indecisiveness
- Injuries not requiring surgery
- Insomnia
- Irritable bowel syndrome (IBS)
- Jaw tension
- Joint pain
- Learning difficulties
- Low self-esteem
- Menstrual disorders
- Migraine
- Mood swings
- Muscle strain
- Muscular aches and pains
- Nausea
- Neck ache and stiffness
- Nervous problems
- Neuralgia
- Phobias
- Post-operative pain
- Postural imbalances
- Pre-menstrual syndrome (PMS)
- Restlessness
- Sciatica
- Sinusitis
- Skin disorders
- Sports injuries
- Stage-fright
- Stress
- Sub-fertility
- Tennis elbow
- Tinnitus
- TMJ (Temporomandibular joint) jaw problems
- Weight problems (over and under)

As can be seen, Kinesiology can be helpful with many common conditions which orthodox medicine may alleviate but not necessarily cure. All the conditions listed have been effectively dealt with using the Kinesiology approach of assessing all aspects of the person and correcting the imbalances found, rather than by directly treating symptoms.

To take just one example, more and more people today are suffering from Chronic Fatigue Syndrome, widely known as M.E. (Myalgic Encephalomyelitis, which is really something of a misnomer). Although the condition is now generally recognized by medical doctors, its cause remains a mystery, and few GPs can offer much help other than to recommend plenty of rest. By investigating all aspects of the sufferer, the Kinesiologist can recommend the most appropriate diet, and help to deal with stress and any other unhelpful elements of the person's lifestyle. Most importantly, correcting imbalances in the subtle energy system has the effect of raising the sufferer's depleted energy levels and lifting him or her out of the despair caused by low energy (see Chapter 8).

IS KINESIOLOGY SAFE?

When practised by people who are properly trained, Kinesiology cannot harm anyone. The techniques used for correction are simple and gentle; they work by enhancing the client's energy, following the dictates of the client's own body as to what is energy-enhancing and what is not.

Any therapy is only as good as the person practising it, and there is, it should be said, a danger of some apparently simple techniques being picked up and practised by untrained people. Unfortunately, the freedom of alternative therapists to practise in some countries, including Britain, has its abusers. It has been known for people to visit so-called Kinesiologists and to be told after minimal testing that they have a serious illness, or must live on nothing but rice cakes because they have multiple allergies. Conversely, serious conditions can be missed by someone who sets up as a therapist after doing a weekend workshop in muscle testing.

Muscle testing will be described fully in Chapter 4; it is an art, and to do it reliably and expertly requires good training and practice. Anyone can say, 'Hold out your arm' and then press on it. This is not Kinesiology muscle testing. Unfortunately, however, many therapists do this, and claim they are using Kinesiology or even Applied Kinesiology. But unless the practitioner is aware of the many factors that can affect a muscle test, his or her conclusions may be inaccurate.

It must be stressed that properly-trained Kinesiologists do not aim or claim to give a medical diagnosis, unless they are qualified to do so. Most people visiting a Kinesiologist for the first time with a medical condition will already have had a diagnosis from their GP, and if not, will be advised by the Kinesiologist to do so.

KINESIOLOGY AS PREVENTION

The ideal use for Kinesiology is in preventive health care, to keep the physical, emotional and energy systems in balance so that problems are less likely to arise. Used in this way, in conjunction with self-help techniques (described in Chapter 6), it can help people to achieve and maintain optimum health.

Moreover, Kinesiology can detect imbalances *before* they develop into physical symptoms and disease. This is particularly true when the muscle-meridian connections and Meridian Therapy are used for assessment and treatment.

Today, the importance of the human energy systems, including the meridians within the body and the energy field around

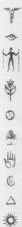

it, is recognized within several branches of medicine, increasingly grouped together as 'energy medicine' or 'vibrational medicine'. Energy medicine includes homoeopathy, healing, the Bach Flower Remedies and, of course, acupuncture. As Dr Richard Gerber puts it, 'The acupuncture meridian system is an interface of energetic exchange between our physical body and the energy fields which surround us.' (Richard Gerber, *Vibrational Medicine: New Choices for Healing Ourselves*, Santa Fe, NM: Bear & Co., 1988, page 189.)

It is widely accepted among practitioners of energy medicine that health problems appear first in the subtle body, or subtle energy fields, before materializing in the physical body. The subtle energy body – referred to by some healers as the *aura* – consists of a series of energy fields surrounding the physical body. Invisible to most people, these fields can be seen and felt by sensitives such as healers, who are often able to foresee a health problem before the person concerned is aware of it.

Kinesiology is one way of enabling practitioners to detect potential problems in the subtle energy field. By obtaining a read-out of the meridians through muscle testing, a Kinesiologist can discover subtle energy imbalances that are having, or are about to have, an effect on the physical body, which in time could lead to symptoms and disease.

A fairly typical example is the client who comes to a Kinesiologist complaining of tiredness, mood swings, disorientation, and a range of other rather vague symptoms. On testing, the Kinesiologist finds that the latissimus dorsi muscle (a large muscle in the back) is weak. This muscle is connected to the spleen meridian, which energizes the pancreas, the gland that produces insulin and controls blood-sugar levels. On questioning the client, the Kinesiologist discovers that the client has a craving for sugar.

The Kinesiologist will use the appropriate corrections to strengthen the weak muscle; further testing confirms that the muscle has been strengthened, which indicates that energy has been restored to the spleen meridian and its associated gland, the pancreas. To maintain this, the client will be advised to reduce his or her sugar intake and increase consumption of foods rich in Vitamin A.

Had the imbalance in the pancreas gland been severe, and allowed to continue undetected and untreated over a long period, the client could have developed diabetes.

Touch For Health is, of course, specifically designed for prevention, and can usefully be learned by anyone who wants to help maintain his or her family's health.

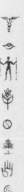

VISITS TO A KINESIOLOGIST

When you decide to try Kinesiology treatment for yourself, there are a number of factors to take into account: who is available, what branch do they practise, and with what other therapies or skills do they combine it?

Although Kinesiology is practised extensively in the USA, this is not the case in every country, and you may not be able to find a Kinesiologist on your doorstep. However, the field is expanding, and more and more people are training in Kinesiology all the time.

While TFH and AK form the foundation of all Kinesiology, many branches have developed that focus on different areas of health care, each with its specialized methods of assessment and correction. The main branches are described in Chapter 7. Their variety shows the wealth of possibilities offered by Kinesiology.

As well as each branch offering its specialist approach, most Kinesiologists combine Kinesiology with some other therapy, such as counselling, nutrition, osteopathy, chiropractic and other forms of body work. So although Kinesiology may form the main basis of their work, individual practitioners will have different approaches based both on the branch they practise and the other skills they use.

Appendix B includes a list of contact people for the different branches and applications of Kinesiology, who will be able to refer you to your nearest practitioner.

The choice can be somewhat bewildering, however. How should you decide which one is right for you?

CHOOSING A KINESIOLOGIST

The ideal is to choose a Kinesiologist who has the combination of skills that meets your needs. If, for example, you have a back problem, your first choice might be an osteopath or chiropractor who uses Kinesiology. Alternatively, you could also get an assessment from a Kinesiologist who is not a manipulative therapist, and if the problem were muscular, as is often the case, he or she might well be able to correct it. However, if it was found that you needed manipulation, you would be referred to a chiropractor or osteopath.

If, on the other hand, you are suffering from emotional stress, your needs might be better met by going to a Kinesiologist who specializes in emotional issues; while if you have a nutritional or allergy problem a nutritionist using Kinesiology techniques will be able to assess your dietary requirements.

Since there are so many ways of using Kinesiology, it is important to find someone who not only has the skills you require but also works in a way that feels comfortable to you. In practice, your choice may be limited by who is available locally. Whatever the variations, most practitioners will have had a basic training in Touch For Health. Whoever you go to, it is advisable to state that you wish the first session to be a consultation, with no commitment at that stage to ongoing treatment.

To help you find your way around what could be a confusing picture, there is a summary chart on page 132 showing the different focus of each system or branch of Kinesiology.

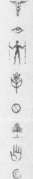

FEES

Professional Kinesiologists, like other therapists, have to charge for their services. Fees are determined by a number of factors: training, experience, duration of the sessions, and location (overheads in big cities, for instance, are usually higher than they are elsewhere).

The holistic approach adopted by most Kinesiologists can be time-consuming, and sessions involving Kinesiology can be longer than those without. However, Kinesiology can usually get to the cause of the problem quickly, even when other systems have failed, and the correction techniques are fast and effective. So, although individual sessions can be longer and therefore more costly than those of some other therapies, there will usually be fewer visits and longer-lasting results.

THE FIRST SESSION

The session described in this chapter is based on the typical practice of a professional Kinesiologist using the holistic model of AK/TFH. The duration of sessions varies considerably. An osteopath or chiropractor might see you for 30 minutes the first time and 15 minutes at subsequent sessions. Almost all other Kinesiologists give sessions lasting an hour or longer.

Much of the first session will be spent in gathering information. Whatever your specific problems, the practitioner will be building up a picture of the balance of your structural, nutritional and emotional states, and energy factors.

TAKING A CASE HISTORY

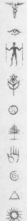

The Kinesiologist will start by taking a case history: asking questions about your current symptoms, and any medical diagnosis and treatment, together with your medical history including illnesses, operations and medical treatment. He or she will also want to know something about your lifestyle, including exercise and relaxation, stresses, diet, relationships, and your home and working life.

X-rays

Chiropractors and osteopaths sometimes require X-rays (some take their own); if so, it is worth finding out whether any existing X-rays can be obtained before having new ones taken.

Medical Diagnosis

The Kinesiologist will ask you whether you have seen your GP, and may advise you to do so. Unless he or she is qualified to give a medical diagnosis, the Kinesiology assessment provides an *energy* assessment of various parts of the body and body functions. If, having seen your doctor, the medical diagnosis suggests that you require treatment, you may discuss the most appropriate treatment with your Kinesiologist – orthodox medicine, Kinesiology, or a combination of the two. It is always worth seeing what can be done before having any surgery, as you can't replace parts once they have been surgically removed, nor can you eliminate scar tissue once it is there.

It could happen that during the assessment the Kinesiologist may suspect the presence of a health problem of which you are unaware, warranting medical investigation. In this case the Kinesiologist would refer you to your GP. This is often only precautionary, but nevertheless should be heeded, as the following story shows.

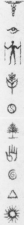

SEVERE SINUS PROBLEMS

A man came to see me suffering from severe sinus problems, which he had had for years. He had seen his doctor about a year before, but had decided that he wanted to be healed 'naturally', and had tried various natural therapies.

During the assessment I realized that he might have a more serious problem than he thought. I advised him to see his GP again, and to ask for a referral to an Ear, Nose and Throat specialist before proceeding with Kinesiology treatment.

He took my advice, and a week later was undergoing surgery for a suspected cancerous growth. Fortunately he had the operation in time; the growth turned out to be pre-cancerous.

Such dramatic cases are, fortunately, very rare.

KINESIOLOGY ASSESSMENT

Once the case history has been taken the assessment will be carried out. The Kinesiologist will pay attention to any specific symptoms you have, but because Kinesiology is based on an holistic model, the assessment will cover all aspects – structural, chemical and emotional, and also electromagnetic. Giving attention to all these areas often reveals the underlying or hidden causes of symptoms.

Muscle Testing

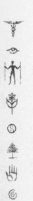

Using the standard AK/TFH assessment methods, the Kinesiologist will perform a series of muscle tests on both sides of your body to assess the energy balance of the muscles, meridians and related organs and glands. He or she will also perform one test, called an indicator muscle test, to assess a whole range of other factors. These techniques are described more fully in Chapter 4.

Unless the Kinesiologist is also a manipulative therapist, such as an osteopath or chiropractor, you will not have to undress; testing can be done fully clothed. You may be asked to remove some clothing in later sessions, so that the Kinesiologist can better analyse your posture for muscle imbalance.

Most muscle tests are performed while you are lying down on a treatment couch, which makes it easier to test your leg muscles. A few of the tests involve movements for which you will be asked to stand.

While you are lying comfortably, the Kinesiologist will move your arm into a particular position and then instruct you to 'hold' while he or she applies light pressure on the arm in a particular direction for a couple of seconds. This is to find out whether or not the muscle being tested can lock instantly in position.

The Kinesiologist will then proceed with a series of muscle tests on both sides of your body, each time placing your arm or leg in a different position – none of them uncomfortable – and each time applying light pressure for a few seconds.

You will find that while some muscles lock effortlessly, others give way when tested. This can be quite a surprise, since we are not normally aware of these minor muscle weaknesses. For example, many right-handed people assume that their right arm is the stronger, and are surprised if this doesn't prove to be the case. However, the purpose of this process is not to test your strength but to evaluate the quality of your muscle response and the energy immediately available to it.

Corrections

Although most of this first session is likely to be spent information-gathering, you will receive some corrections during the assessment. These are mostly painless, and the results instantaneous. Some of them are described more fully in Chapters 5 and 6. It is important to know that the more information the Kinesiologist can gather through assessment, the more precise and effective the corrections or treatment will be.

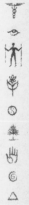

Summary of Assessment

At the end of the first session, the Kinesiologist will be able to give you a summary of the main areas of imbalance that your body has shown, citing specific imbalances and the possible connections between your symptoms and his or her findings. You may also be told about the corrections you have been given. You may be advised to attend weekly for three to four sessions, and then at less frequent intervals as your symptoms disappear.

EFFECTS OF A KINESIOLOGY SESSION

Most people find Kinesiology treatment very relaxing, and some feel pleasantly lighter and more 'clear' afterwards. However, because treatments are powerful and deep-reaching, they can bring about major energy changes, resulting in temporary feelings of tiredness or sleepiness, or other slight symptoms. This is actually a good sign, and should not cause you any concern: it is an indication that your body is going through a healing process. It is best helped by resting or sleeping; in fact, it is worth planning your appointment with the Kinesiologist to allow yourself enough time to rest afterwards. Although the energy changes occur instantly at the time when treatment is given, the healing effects can continue for days, weeks, and even months following treatment.

The body has the innate ability to heal itself, and it does this quite naturally; for instance, if you cut your finger, it will automatically heal itself in time. Kinesiology, by balancing all aspects of the person – structural, chemical and mental – puts the body in an optimum state for self-healing. How long this takes will, of course, depend on the individual.

After your first visit it is up to you to decide whether you wish to return for follow-up sessions, and you are free to decide this in your own time.

Although the procedures for each session are similar, no two will be exactly the same. Each time one imbalance is corrected, another imbalance will appear as a priority; that is, as the next correction the body needs. This process continues until all the imbalances have been corrected and the body is finally in balance.

For example, the Kinesiologist may start by correcting a structural priority, such as some weak muscles; once this has been cleared, your body may then show that an emotional issue or chemical imbalance needs to be addressed, or even possibly another structural one. Sometimes all or the major part of a session may be devoted to testing for allergies and sensitivities, as this takes time. As the Kinesiologist deals with each aspect and strengthens one side of the Triad, this will support changes in the other sides.

An example is the woman with the milk allergy described in Chapter 1. The first treatment cleared her headache, but the return of the muscle weakness showed a chemical priority. This was related to an allergy which, on testing, turned out to be to milk. When the chemical problem was cleared by cutting out milk, an emotional priority emerged.

As treatment progresses, fewer imbalances are present, and usually all will eventually disappear. Meanwhile you will feel progressively better.

DURATION OF TREATMENT

Because Kinesiology is such an effective system, it is not usually necessary to attend many sessions before experiencing an improvement; it is reasonable to expect a noticeable improvement

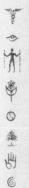

by at least the third session. Indeed, some clients have commented on the extraordinary speed with which corrections take effect. Corrections are in fact instantaneous, although it can take time for you to experience the results of the change that they have brought about. People often ask: 'How long does the benefit last?' The answer is that it lasts until some stress factor recurs to cause an imbalance. The Kinesiologist's task is to discover these stress factors and re-educate the body to accept a new state of balance.

However, Kinesiology is not a magic wand, and it is important to distinguish between short-term problems, which can be dealt with in a couple of sessions, and chronic problems, which may require considerably longer treatment. Healing is an ongoing process that may take days, weeks or even months to complete, as in the following case.

A LONG-TERM HEALING PROCESS

A 48-year-old man came to see me complaining of a very swollen eyelid, which he had suffered from for six months. An eye specialist had been unable to identify the cause of the problem; it was relieved, but not cured, by cortisone cream.

On talking with him, it became clear that although he had no current emotional stress, he had a history of loss and grief. The assessment showed that the eye problem was related to a weak kidney meridian, and general toxicity. The man also suffered from constipation, and his diet was poor. He drank up to six cups of strong coffee daily, and had only recently given up smoking. His system was sluggish and toxic, having suffered from the ongoing stimulation of cigarettes and coffee for many years.

This was not going to be a quick, overnight cure. I stimulated the man's lymphatic and meridian systems, and gave him some dietary recommendations and daily exercises to do. I also worked with him on the emotional issues, and he came to realize that he could make some changes in his lifestyle that would generate and stimulate new interests.

The man came for six treatments at monthly intervals, at the same time following up my recommendations about self-help. In the short-term, there was an improvement in the eye condition and in his general health, and his attitude to life became more positive. At the end of the treatment, the eye condition had completely cleared up.

The man is now much fitter, and has a new and important interest in his life. He continues to visit me from time to time for maintenance.

SELF-HELP

One of the many benefits of Kinesiology is that you actively participate in the session; you partake in the muscle testing and can experience for yourself, for instance, how weak muscles become strong after corrections, or the effects on your system of milk, sugar or coffee, or of your beliefs and attitudes, without having to take the practitioner's views on trust.

Participation can also continue between sessions. The Kinesiologist may recommend a change in diet, and can test how effective this has been at the next session. Or self-help may be suggested, in the form of exercises, self-massage of reflex points, or using the emotional stress release technique. (Some of these self-help techniques are described in Chapter 6.)

MAINTENANCE

The analogy of maintenance with looking after a car may sound amusing, but there are some similarities. You don't expect your car to go on running for years without having it checked over, and possibly having some minor repairs. Your

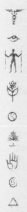

body is much the same. It can benefit from a regular check-up and minor repairs when necessary, to keep it functioning well. Many people who have experienced Kinesiology acknowledge this, and go for regular energy balancing as a form of maintenance. What's more, you don't need to be unwell to qualify for energy balancing or maintenance. Many fit, healthy people include it as part of their fitness programme.

KEEPING HEALTHY WITH TOUCH FOR HEALTH

It may also be possible for you to have a Kinesiology session with a friend who has learned Touch For Health and would like to share this with you on a non-professional basis. Many more people throughout the world have experienced Kinesiology from friends than from professional Kinesiology practitioners. Touch For Health offers a wide range of gentle energy-balancing techniques, and many people who have no professional involvement or background in health care use these techniques very effectively. If you are healthy – not suffering from a specific disease or illness – a Touch For Health balance from a friend or relative can be a wonderful experience. As John Thie says, 'All you need is a loving pair of hands.'

KINESIOLOGY
ASSESSMENT

Kinesiology offers one of the most effective methods of assessment available in natural health care today.

Through the use of muscle testing, the Kinesiologist can gain information about almost any part of the body, and about the body's response to any stimulus. This chapter describes the various factors that can be assessed, and the range of techniques used, most of which are unique to Kinesiology; it will help you to understand more about the treatments described in the case histories given later.

DIFFERENT TYPES OF ASSESSMENT

AK ASSESSMENT

AK assesses six major factors, any of which can cause muscle weakness and accompanying organ malfunction. One is a chemical imbalance related to nutrition; the others are structural problems, and are known as the five factors of the IVF (intervertebral foramen). The IVF is the space or hole in the side of each vertebra (the bones that make up the spine) through which nerves, blood vessels and lymphatic vessels come out from the spinal cord into the rest of the body. If there is any imbalance in the structural, chemical or emotional aspects of the person, this will manifest as muscle weakness, and one of these five factors will be functioning abnormally. The five factors are:

1. Subluxation (jamming or misalignment of the vertebrae)
2. Lymphatic congestion
3. Vascular (circulatory) stagnation
4. Dural torque CSF (a twist in the dura mater, the sheath around the spinal cord, affecting the flow of cerebro-spinal fluid)
5. Acupuncture/meridian imbalance

AK tests more muscles, and more precise parts of muscles, than does TFH.

TFH ASSESSMENT

Whereas AK, coming from a chiropractic background, uses structural assessment and manipulation, the non-manipulative TFH system places greater emphasis on energy balancing and other factors, including the emotions.

TFH assesses up to 42 major muscles in the body. As in an AK assessment, any imbalance in the structural, chemical or emotional aspects of the person will show up as muscle weakness. But because TFH does not include manipulation, the assessment does not include subluxations, but seeks to find out whether the muscle weakness is due to lymphatic congestion, vascular stagnation, acupuncture or meridian imbalance, faulty muscle programming, and/or nutritional or emotional problems.

ASSESSMENT WITHOUT MUSCLE TESTING

As part of the initial assessment, a Kinesiologist who practises energy balancing may use some non-muscle testing methods from the Law of Five Elements, a system within traditional Chinese medicine, used by many acupuncturists today. This relates everything on earth, and in the body, to one of five elements: fire, earth, metal, water or wood, all of which interact with each other. According to this philosophy, health comes from being in harmony with the five elements, which are linked to the meridians and the main body organs (see chart page 64).

The Kinesiologist can use this system to place his or her findings about muscles and meridians within the context of the Five Elements. Each element relates to a specific emotion, colour, sound, smell, taste (e.g. sweet, bitter, etc.), and season. In assessment these connections are used, for example, by noting the client's skin colour, tone of voice, body odour, favourite foods and preferred time of year, all of which have a particular meaning in terms of meridian balance and health. This information, combined with other details gained through muscle testing, gives the practitioner a very rich and comprehensive picture of the client's present state.

WHAT CAN BE ASSESSED?

Although the factors that can be assessed are almost limitless, this chapter describes those that are commonly assessed in AK/TFH and some branches of Kinesiology. Kinesiology organizes these factors into the general categories of structural, chemical, emotional and electrical (a Summary Chart is given on page 47.

STRUCTURAL FACTORS

Structural factors include the muscles and bones; an imbalance in these can cause poor posture, pain or discomfort. Kinesiology tests the major muscles of the body to identify those that are weak and those that are tight, as well as testing

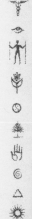

44 for subluxations, misalignments or jamming of the bones of the spine, the cranium (skull) and the pelvis. Other structural tests include testing the shock absorbers in the ankles, knees and thighs, testing for hiatus hernia, and checking the ileocecal valve (ICV).

The ICV is found at the junction of the small and large intestines. If this valve is not working properly – that is, if it is too open, or too closed – it can give rise to a whole range of seemingly unrelated problems such as headaches, constipation, diarrhoea and Candida Albicans. (Candida, also called Candidiasis, is a yeast overgrowth which has only recently been recognized, mainly in the alternative health field, as being the cause of a number of symptoms such as bloating, vaginal discharge, mental confusion, nausea, irritable bowel syndrome, etc.)

CHEMICAL FACTORS

Chemical factors include allergic reactions, nutritional deficiencies, hormonal imbalances, blood-sugar imbalances and toxicity. These upset the body chemistry and can give rise to a wide range of symptoms such as mental confusion, skin conditions, headaches and dizziness, and Candida, to name but a few.

Kinesiology offers perhaps the most effective and accurate method of testing for allergies and sensitivities to food and other substances. Unlike most other methods of allergy testing, it is immediate and painless. It uses the body's own response to test for reactions to foods, liquids and airborne and tactile allergens such as cat fur and moulds, metal toxicity (e.g. mercury), environmental and geopathic stress, alcohol, tobacco, and food supplements. Kinesiology can also distinguish between a full-blown allergic reaction and a sensitivity, and thus between the need to avoid something altogether or just to reduce exposure to it.

Emotional factors include our thoughts, beliefs, attitudes and feelings, both conscious and unconscious, relating to the past, present and future – all of which can cause a range of mental and emotional problems including stress, anxiety, insomnia, addictions and phobias. These emotional factors not only have an effect on our behaviour, they also have a profound effect on all aspects of our health. You become what you believe, and what you are now is the sum of what you have believed and thought about in the past. So in dealing with any health problem it is important to identify any emotional factors that may be involved.

Muscle testing gives an instant, non-verbal body response – an unconscious response – to emotional stimuli. It can reveal the inner conflicts and hidden negative beliefs and attitudes that are often involved in addictions, wherein people find themselves sabotaging the positive changes that consciously they wish to make. The Kinesiology test for this is called 'psychological reversal' (see page 85). Muscle testing can elicit precise information about emotional issues: for example, exactly when a problem started, where, and with whom, which can be helpful in dealing with all kinds of difficulties, including anxieties and phobias, and with identifying the emotional factors often entailed in allergies. It can also identify the stress that often gets locked in the body at the time of an accident or trauma, giving rise to chronic pain.

ELECTROMAGNETIC FACTORS

These encompass a number of energy circuits in the body and energy fields extending to within 2 in/5 cm around the body. Electromagnetic problems are caused by electrical disturbances in these systems which create poor or faulty communication within the body, often giving rise to feelings of disorientation and confusion, poor co-ordination, dyslexia, etc. Tranquillizers and other drugs, medical and social, can be major causes of electromagnetic imbalance.

Electromagnetic factors include:

- *Ionization:* that is, the balance of positive and negative ions that we breathe in, which create positive and negative currents within the body
- *Centring:* that is, how the body responds to instant shock. Centring includes right-/left-brain dominance, gait or walking energy circuits, and cranial/sacral motion
- *Polarity switching:* the body is like a battery, with positive and negative poles (see page 96)
- *Acupuncture meridians (energy pathways):* Kinesiology assesses 14 meridians for over- and under-energy, each relating to a specific part or parts of the body, including:
  The brain and the spine
  Organs: stomach, spleen, heart, lungs, liver, gall-bladder, kidneys, bladder, small intestine, large intestine
  Glands: pancreas, thyroid, adrenals, reproductive glands, thymus
- *Right-/left-brain hemisphere integration:* In most people the left hemisphere of the brain specializes in processing information sequentially, or logically and analytically, in small chunks of information, whereas the right hemisphere perceives spatial concepts, patterns, rhythms, music, etc. as a whole. (In some people these sides are reversed.) Each hemisphere controls the opposite side of the body, so poor integration of the hemispheres affects both mental functioning and the physical body. When the two are not integrated, a person can get stuck in one mode of thinking; for example, someone with an over-dominant analytical hemisphere may only be able to think of the logical outcome of a problem, and

unable to think laterally to find a solution. Hemisphere imbalance can also be a key factor in dyslexia, learning difficulties and poor co-ordination.

- *Visual inhibition:* i.e. an assessment of the energy circuits relating to the eyes. (This was relevant in the case of the little boy in Chapter 2.)
- *Auricular* i.e. the energy circuits related to the ears.

SUMMARY CHART OF WHAT CAN BE ASSESSED IN AK/TFH AND SOME BRANCHES OF KINESIOLOGY

Structural factors *Muscles:* In TFH 42 major muscles on both sides of the body, in the arms, hands, legs, ankles, front of torso, back of torso and neck, are tested. In AK more muscles are tested, more specifically.

Bones: The vertebrae of the spine, the cranium (skull) and pelvis. Other areas tested include the shock absorbers in the ankles, knees and hips; the teeth; the ileoceoal valve; hiatal hernia.

Chemical factors Allergies to foods, liquids, or airborne and tactile substances; toxicity, nutritional deficiencies, hormonal and blood-sugar imbalances.

Emotional factors Feelings of all kinds, beliefs, attitudes, conscious and unconscious, relating to the past, present and future, inner conflicts (psychological reversal).

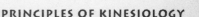

PRINCIPLES OF KINESIOLOGY

Electromagnetic factors

Energy circuits in the body and energy fields within 2 in/5 cm of the body.

Ionization, centring (R/L brain dominance, gait or walking circuits, cranial/sacral motion). Polarity switching and R/L brain integration.

Energy circuits relating to the eyes and ears. Brain and spine.

Organs: Stomach, spleen, heart, lungs, liver, gall-bladder, kidneys, bladder, small intestine, large intestine.

Glands: Pancreas, thyroid, adrenals, reproductive glands, thymus.

ASSESSMENT METHODS

MUSCLE TESTING

Muscle testing is the principal method of assessment used in Kinesiology, and it is the use of muscle testing that distinguishes Kinesiology from all other therapies. There are a number of different ways of using muscle testing in assessment.

There is nothing new about the manual testing of muscles; physiotherapists often use it to assess the strength of specific muscles, particularly in patients who have a weakness as a result of, say, poliomyelitis, a stroke or an injury. Physiotherapists evaluate muscle strength against gravity on a scale of 0–5, 0 being equivalent to no response and 5 to normal strength.

Most muscles tested on this 0–5 scale fall within the 5 range. However, many of these 'normal' muscles would fail a Kinesiology muscle test, which assesses the *quality* of the muscle response, which is determined by the nervous system. In this Kinesiology is unique.

In Kinesiology muscle testing, the muscle to be tested is isolated as far as possible from the other muscles with which it normally works. It is put into contraction – that is, the two ends of the muscle are brought closer together. The person being tested is asked to hold that position, while the testor applies light pressure, about 2 lbs/1 kg or less, for about two seconds, pushing in a direction that will extend the muscle. If the limb moves more than 2 in/5 cm it is considered weak; if it holds, it is strong.

Isolating the muscle in this way makes it more difficult for the person to maintain the starting position of the test. It tests the ability of the person's nervous system to adapt to the changing pressure of the testor during the two-second period. This allows the testor to evaluate the muscle response.

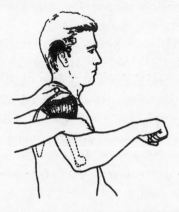

Figure 1: Kinesiology muscle testing (deltoid muscle test)

TWO METHODS OF USING MUSCLE TESTING

The method of testing a muscle from contraction to extension is the same throughout all branches of Kinesiology. Muscle testing is a form of muscle biofeedback, in that the strong or weak response gives the testor specific information.

In Kinesiology assessment, muscle testing is used in two different ways:

1. As a series of specific muscle tests, to find out how well the body is functioning in all aspects – structural, chemical, emotional and energetic.
2. With an indicator muscle (IM) test, which uses a single muscle to get a non-verbal response to a stimulus, which could be structural, chemical, emotional or electromagnetic.

All branches of Kinesiology use both methods, and some branches make greater use of the indicator muscle test.

The Indicator Muscle (IM) Test

This involves using one muscle only as a biofeedback tool to gain information about the body/mind or any of its parts *other than* the specific muscle being tested.

A muscle used in this way is called an indicator muscle (IM). It can be any muscle in the body which is strong and functioning normally; its association with a meridian in this case is not important. This single muscle can be used to test the body's response to a stimulus, and it will weaken under light pressure when the stimulus is causing disorganization or imbalance in the client's system. For example, if the Cross Crawl exercise (described on page 73) causes stress in the system, a previously strong IM will weaken.

It is thought that the reason for this is that, if the muscle is strong and there is no stress, the brain can cope simultaneously with the muscle test and the additional, non-stressful stimulus. If, however, the stimulus causes some stress, this creates a momentary disorganization in the brain, which cannot cope with two stressors simultaneously – i.e. keeping the muscle strong and dealing with the effect of the stimulus. The brain prioritizes the stress and as a result, the indicator muscle instantly weakens.

In AK and Touch For Health an indicator muscle test is always used in conjunction with other assessment techniques as a means of assessing structure, chemistry, emotions and electromagnetic energy. However, some branches of Kinesiology make extensive use of an IM test on its own to assess emotional factors and to get 'yes/strong' or 'no/weak' responses to verbal questions. This is sometimes referred to as 'asking the body', or 'intuitive muscle testing'.

Uses and Abuses of Indicator Muscle Testing

Indicator muscle testing can appear quite dramatic; it opens up the amazing possibility of testing the body's response immediately to almost anything. It is this tremendous scope for muscle biofeedback that has led to the rapid expansion of Kinesiology into so many different fields of health care.

As mentioned earlier, however, this technique must be carried out by properly-trained practitioners. A number of factors can affect a muscle test, and lacking an awareness of these the testor can come up with erroneous information. Its use in 'asking the body' must also be treated with care, as not all Kinesiologists can use this method reliably all the time.

'Asking the Body' – Is it Reliable?

There is a broad divide between Kinesiologists who use AK-based methods of assessment and those who 'ask the body'. AK Practitioners, with its more scientific and medically-orientated

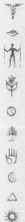

background, use a logical, non-intuitive method of assessment to access information from the body. Those who use the method of 'asking the body' trust in a more intuitive process of tapping directly into the body's wisdom.

There are advantages and disadvantages in both methods. AK, by defining what can be assessed and how, limits the potential scope of assessment, particularly in the area of the emotions; however, the results of the AK method can be replicated. 'Asking the body' gives unlimited scope for assessment of all kinds of factors, but because it depends more on intuition it produces results that are not always repeatable, and are consequently less reliable. Nevertheless, in experienced and skilled hands, 'asking the body' can lead to quite remarkable results, as some of the case histories in Chapter 7 demonstrate.

The reason 'asking the body' may not be reliable, however, seems to be that if the practitioner is not totally detached, he or she can interact with the person as a surrogate and thus influence the outcome of the test, albeit unintentionally. To quote David Walther, one of the leading authorities and writers on AK: 'It appears that some individuals can apply apparent therapeutic approaches and obtain results that cannot be accomplished by others ... these procedures may be valuable to that individual, but they cannot be taught to others who may not have the same capabilities and mental matrices.' (David S. Walther, DC, *Applied Kinesiology*, Systems DC, USA, 1981, vol 1, page 5.)

Practitioners, students and clients tend to select the approach with which they feel most comfortable.

FURTHER ASSESSMENT TECHNIQUES

There are a number of further techniques to gain even more information from the body/mind. These are unique to

Kinesiology and are used in conjunction with either specific muscle tests or an indicator muscle test.

Some systems and branches of Kinesiology use some of these techniques and not others, while some use them in combination. There are slight variations in their definitions.

Therapy Localizing (TL)

This procedure is used for testing structural, chemical and electromagnetic energy factors, in order to find out exactly where a problem lies. The Kinesiologist tests an indicator muscle while the client touches the suspected area – perhaps a part of the skull, an acupuncture point or a particular tooth. If the previously strong indicator muscle weakens, this indicates an imbalance in the part of the body being touched. Therapy Localizing – or circuit locating, as it is sometimes called – can also be used to find the location of a treatment that will change a weak muscle response to a strong one.

Challenging

This procedure is the same as the one for Therapy Localizing, but it is the practitioner who touches the point or points in question, for example to find out which vertebra is out of alignment.

Challenging is also the name given to a technique used to indicate whether the specific treatment just given is enough, or whether another kind of treatment is also required.

Two-pointing

In this procedure the Kinesiologist tests a muscle while two problem areas are touched simultaneously (either by the practitioner or the client), to find out whether there is a connection between the two, for example between the base of the skull and the lower back. There is often an important connection, as is illustrated in the case history on page 54.

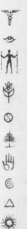

Therapy Localizing, Challenging and Two-pointing are used extensively in AK, and in some (but not all) branches of Kinesiology.

Prioritizing

One of the most important and unique diagnostic tools in Kinesiology is the ability to *prioritize* problems or imbalances: that is, to identify the primary problem as distinct from secondary ones. This was introduced by Dr Sheldon Deal.

If your lights go out because a fuse has blown, fiddling with individual light fittings won't put the lights on again. To restore all the lights on that circuit, the source of the primary problem in the fusebox must be found and mended. The body is rather similar: identify the primary problem, and a number of secondary ones will automatically clear up.

During assessment, prioritizing is used to identify the primary as distinct from the secondary problems. Corrections are then focused on the primary problems. Below is an example of how useful Therapy Localizing, Challenging, Two-pointing and prioritizing can be in tracking down the primary cause of a serious medical problem, which would otherwise have been treated with unnecessary major surgery.

LOWER BACK PAIN AND A CRANIAL PROBLEM

One of my clients had a serious problem in her lower back affecting the lumbar vertebrae (technically known as L4 and L5), and had suffered chronic pain for over 15 years. When she came to see me, she was on a waiting list for a spinal fusion operation.

The Kinesiology assessment confirmed through Challenging that she had a lower back problem. However, Therapy Localizing also indicated that some of her cranial bones – the bones that form the skull – were jammed; normally they should be very slightly movable. Two-pointing revealed a connection between the two. (The importance of this particular connection is recognized by the increasing number of osteopaths and chiropractors these days who use cranial or cranio-sacral therapy, gentle methods of treating the head, jaw, and lower back.)

Further testing showed that this cranial problem took priority over the woman's lower back problem. I referred her to a chiropractor-Kinesiologist for a second opinion and possible treatment. He confirmed the findings of my first assessment, and made an adjustment to the jammed bones of her skull.

Following this treatment her chronic back pain disappeared dramatically, and has never returned. She has not had to have any surgery. She still has a weakness in her back, but with careful management she keeps this under control and is pain-free for most of the time.

Hand/finger Modes

A further development in assessment procedures has been the introduction of hand and other modes, developed in Clinical Kinesiology (CK, see page 125), and of 'finger modes' as developed in PKP (see page 106). These modes involve the practitioner or the client putting his or her fingers into particular configurations which may then make a strong muscle go weak, or a weak muscle go strong. Hand modes provide a kind of nonverbal language with which the practitioner can ask questions about connections between different factors, appropriate treatments, and priorities. This is a highly complex system, using a vocabulary of hundreds of hand modes. These modes are not accepted as part of the International College of Applied Kinesiology (ICAK) material.

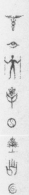

Pause Lock (Circuit Retaining Mode)

This was also developed in CK. It is used to lock information about a specific problem into the whole body. An imbalance is activated, such as a weak muscle, and at the same time the client's legs are rotated outwards and spread about 18 in/45 cm apart. This action transfers the specific problem into the body as a whole, causing every muscle in the body to test weak.

This technique is useful in assessing as it eliminates the need to keep re-testing muscles that are already weak or painful, and facilitates more complex procedures such as muscle reprogramming, two-pointing and prioritizing. It is also used in conjunction with corrections and treatment, to enhance their effect.

Surrogate Testing

When, for whatever reason, the Kinesiologist cannot directly muscle test a person, a surrogate can be used. This technique can be used with very small babies, the elderly, the severely injured, the paralysed, the very sick, the deaf, and even people in a coma. Animals, too, can be assessed in this way.

Surrogate testing includes another person, who agrees to act as a kind of 'energy receiving station' for the person needing help. All the testing is carried out in the normal way on the surrogate, while the surrogate and the client make contact, for example by the client touching the surrogate's shoulder or arm. Effective corrections are also selected in this way. The surrogate does not normally feel any discomfort during this procedure, but people who are very sensitive often feel slight, momentary changes in their own bodies.

It is, of course, essential to test and balance the surrogate beforehand, so that the Kinesiologist is clear that the responses are those of the client and not of the surrogate. Corrections are carried out in the normal way on the person needing help, unless this is physically impossible.

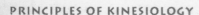

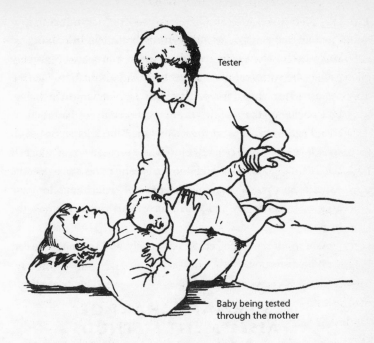

Figure 2: Surrogate testing

Surrogate testing may sound unbelievable, but it works. Although it cannot normally be seen, electromagnetic energy is part of all living systems, including people. When we touch another person, energy is transmitted to and received from them.

This can be demonstrated by using a specially-manufactured light bulb operated by a small battery. (At the time of writing these bulbs are unfortunately not on sale in the UK.) When one person touches a contact point on the battery and the other touches the other contact point, nothing happens. But when they also touch each other, for example by holding hands, the light goes on, showing that their electrical energy has completed the circuit.

A client came for Kinesiology treatment after dislocating his collar-bone in a bicycling accident. Collar-bones are not usually set, so the surrounding muscles need to be strong to hold the bone in place while it is repairing itself. He had his arm in a sling, and obviously the muscles in that area could not be tested. A friend agreed to act as surrogate, and the Kinesiologist first of all muscle tested and cleared him. The surrogate then touched the client's good arm, and through testing the surrogate the Kinesiologist was able to find out precisely which muscles were affected by the injury and which corrections would promote the healing process.

As a result the client recovered quickly, and the injury healed with no distortion.

SUMMARY CHART OF ASSESSMENT METHODS

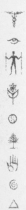

Specific muscle	Series of muscles tests
Indicator muscle test (IM)	In conjunction with other assessment procedures
	On its own as a muscle response to stimuli
	On its own as a muscle response to 'asking the body', 'yes/no'
Therapy Localizing (TL)	Practitioner tests an IM while the client touches a problem area
	or: Practitioner tests a weak muscle while the client touches a treatment point

Challenging	1. The same as for TL but the practitioner touches the problem area as well as testing the muscle 2. A means of indicating whether the specific treatment just given is enough, or if another kind of treatment is required
Two-pointing	The practitioner tests a muscle while two problem areas are touched simultaneously to determine whether there is a connection between the two
Prioritizing	A means of letting the body reveal what is a primary imbalance, which, when corrected, will automatically correct secondary imbalances
Hand/finger modes	Putting the fingers in specific configurations, providing a non-verbal language for asking questions
Circuit retaining mode (pause lock)	As an imbalance is activated, it is locked into the body by rotating the legs outward and spreading them apart
Surrogate testing	Involves an additional person as a surrogate. The person in need of assessment touches the surrogate and the assessment testing is then carried out on the surrogate

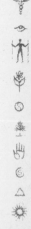

HOW ASSESSMENT IS CARRIED OUT

All Kinesiology assessment is carried out using either specific muscle tests, an indicator muscle test in conjunction with other assessment techniques or movements, or an indicator muscle test in conjunction with a stimulus.

ASSESSING STRUCTURAL FACTORS

Muscles are assessed by the standard muscle testing procedures already described, with specific tests for specific muscles. The vertebrae (the bones of the spine) are assessed by testing an indicator muscle, while the practitioner challenges by touching the bone(s) that may be causing a problem.

Bones in the cranium or skull, including the TMJ (the temporomandibular joint of the jaw), are assessed by testing an indicator muscle while Therapy Localizing, that is with the client touching suspected problem areas.

Not only does muscle testing identify the exact muscle or bone that needs attention, it can also find precisely in which direction the body wants the correction to be made. This very specific information is invaluable to chiropractors and osteopaths when carrying out manipulation, complementing any information they may have gained from X-rays and other assessment procedures.

Hand modes and other modes are also used by some branches of Kinesiology to gain very detailed information about body structure.

ASSESSING CHEMICAL FACTORS
Allergy and Sensitivity
A number of methods are used in allergy testing, and different systems of Kinesiology will use different methods.

In AK/TFH, specific muscle tests are used that are linked closely with the food being tested. For example, the pectoralis major clavicular muscle, located in the upper chest, is connected with the stomach meridian and the stomach, and is involved in the digestion of protein such as milk. If this muscle is strong and then weakens when the person has milk in his or her mouth, this indicates that milk is having a weakening effect on that individual's system – as in the case of the woman with the milk allergy described in Chapter 1.

For allergy testing to be carried out properly and reliably, the Kinesiologist will always test more than one muscle, and will carry out additional tests to distinguish between a sensitivity and an allergy.

Two locations for testing are approved by AK and are also used in Touch For Health. The first is to test the food or substance in the form in which it is normally eaten (i.e. cooked or raw); it is put in the client's mouth and chewed while the relevant muscles are being tested. If this is not appropriate, the substance can be smelled while the tests are being conducted.

You might wonder how testing in the mouth, before the substance is digested, can provide an accurate result. Dr Sheldon Deal explains that '50 per cent of the sensory and motor brain cells are devoted to the TMJ jaw area, i.e. 50 per cent of the brain's messages filter through this area.' (Gordon Stokes and Mary Marks DC, *Dr Sheldon Deal's Basic AK Workshop Manual*, TFH Foundation, 1983, page 42.) This makes the mouth an extremely sensitive area, and as the food or substance mixes with the saliva, messages about the digestive processes are relayed via the brain.

Other locations where the substance can be placed for testing include on or below the navel, near the parotid gland on the cheek, and in the energy field (these locations are not approved by ICAK). Some Kinesiologists perform the test with a homoeopathic potency of the substance enclosed in a glass vial.

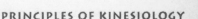

62

It is important to be aware that the Kinesiologist is testing a specific food or substance, rather than testing a general category of food. For example, in assessing a reaction to bread, the response is to the type of bread in the person's mouth, not to all kinds of bread. It is also important to be aware that the result relates to the specific time of assessment, not to yesterday or to next week. So although a practitioner may identify a sensitivity, it is always advisable, before embarking long-term on a restricted diet, to repeat the same test on another day, say three weeks later, to find out whether the reaction was only temporary or whether there is a real ongoing problem.

Getting someone to hold a substance in his or her hand and pressing down on his or her arm without a pre-test is *not* a Kinesiology test. Unfortunately, all too often this method is seen at health fairs and similar places under the banner of Kinesiology.

General Chemical Assessment
Every muscle tested in a Kinesiology assessment not only relates to a part of the body but has associated nutritional factors. That is to say that there are certain nutrients and foods that make each particular muscle strong, others that make it weak, and some that are neutral. So a weak muscle could be an indication of a chemical imbalance. For example, the latissimus dorsi muscle, a large muscle in the back, is connected to the spleen meridian and the pancreas gland, which controls blood-sugar levels. This muscle is tested when assessing the pancreas and its ability to control blood-sugar levels. If this muscle is strong, refined sugar is likely to weaken it.

Nutritional Deficiencies
Another method of assessment (not ICAK-approved) uses nutritional reflexes called Riddlers' reflexes. An indicator muscle is tested while the practitioner touches each of these

reflex points. For example, if a strong indicator muscle weakens when the practitioner touches the reflex point for Vitamin A, which is on the right eyelid, this can be an indication of a Vitamin A deficiency. (This imbalance might also have manifested as a weak muscle, as described on the previous page.)

Nutritional needs change, and should be re-assessed regularly. When the body as a whole is functioning better as a result of energy balancing, it will metabolize food better and will be less likely to have sensitive reactions. This means that someone can show a food sensitivity or nutritional deficiency one month, and possibly not a month later. As Dr Goodheart says, 'You are not what you eat; you are what you *absorb*!'

Some Kinesiologists also use hand modes in chemical assessment.

A nutritional assessment needs to be based on many different factors and should, whenever possible, be considered in conjunction with laboratory tests, not in isolation. There can also be a considerable difference in nutritional needs before and after adjustment of the bones, while certain activities (such as highly demanding sports) or mental states (such as anxiety) require increased nutritional support, which will no longer be needed when these conditions no longer apply.

ASSESSING EMOTIONAL FACTORS

A number of different methods are used in the assessment of emotional factors, and different systems and branches of Kinesiology have their own individual approaches.

In AK/TFH two main methods are used. In the first, two muscles are tested, one related to brain function and one to stomach function. If these test strong but weaken when the person thinks of an emotionally stressful situation, this indicates that this is having a negative or weakening effect on his or her system. This is a non-invasive way of accessing information,

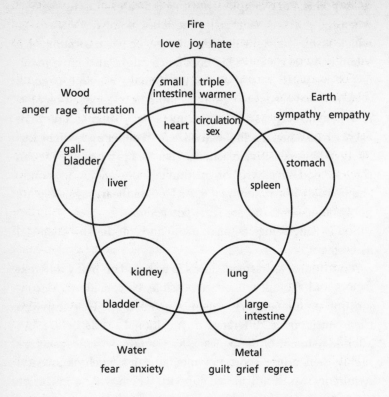

Figure 3: Five Element emotions

since the client does not have to tell the Kinesiologist what he or she is thinking about. If, however, these muscles first test strong but weaken when the person thinks of a positive solution to a problem, and strengthen when he or she thinks of the problem itself, this is an indication of psychological reversal (see page 85) which needs to be corrected before emotional balancing can be effective.

The second assessment method, used by many branches of Kinesiology, draws on the Five Elements (see page 66). Each of the Elements has an emotional aspect. So, since each muscle relates to a meridian, and since each meridian is included in the Law of Five Elements, each muscle also has an emotional component. These connections can help the Kinesiologist to identify emotional factors.

For example, according to this system the liver and gall-bladder are associated with feelings of anger, rage and frustration. So an imbalance in the energy of the muscle related to the liver meridian may be caused by an emotional component such as unexpressed anger – which often turns out to be the case. Experience shows that these correlations can be very accurate.

Some branches of Kinesiology use an IM test, as described on page 50, to assess emotional factors. When a person says, truthfully, 'My name is so-and-so', the muscle will remain strong; if a false name is given, it will weaken. In assessing emotional factors this principle can be used to access information from the unconscious mind, and to identify specific emotions in age regression. For example, the practitioner or client might make the statement, 'The fear of water started between the years 20–15 … 15–10 … 10–5 …' and so on, until the exact age is identified by a change in the muscle response. The IM can also be used to elicit 'Yes' or 'No' responses, while asking, 'Is there an emotional factor? … Is this related to mother? … To father?' … and so on.

Hand modes can also be used in emotional assessment.

ASSESSING ELECTROMAGNETIC FACTORS

Electromagnetic factors are assessed either by an indicator muscle test in conjunction with another assessment technique, by movement or exercise, or by specific muscle tests.

The overall acupuncture energy picture is gained by testing specific muscles which, through the muscle-meridian connection, give information about each meridian. There can be too little meridian energy (under-energy) or an excess of it

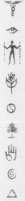

(over-energy). Under-energy is usually identified by weak muscle responses, over-energy by using an IM test while the client touches the pulses on his or her wrists, or specific acupuncture points. This energy information can be understood in terms of the Law of Five Elements, which includes all the meridians and their relationship to each other, and describes predictable patterns of energy movement in the body. Thus, rather than assessing each muscle-meridian imbalance in isolation, imbalances are assessed in relation to each other as part of the whole pattern.

All other electromagnetic factors are tested using the IM test in conjunction with other stimuli such as movement or activating certain points. Many of these tests are described in Chapter 6.

What is assessed	How it is assessed (IM = Indicator Muscle)	
Structure	*Muscles:*	Muscle tested from contraction to extension
	Bones:	Vertebrae: IM and Challenge All other structures use Therapy Localizing (TL) and IM
Chemistry	*Allergies*	AK/TFH test more than one specific muscle with substance in the mouth if appropriate, or smelling it. Plus additional tests. Some branches test food on or below the navel or on the cheek.
	Nutritional deficiencies	Specific muscle tests and IM with nutritional reflexes
	Blood-sugar and hormones	Specific muscle tests
Emotions	AK/TFH: specific muscle tests and The Law of Five Elements (emotional correspondences) Branches use an IM test with 'Asking the Body'	
Electromagnetic factors	All: IM test with specific additional testing procedures (details in Chapter 6)	
	Meridians (and related organs and glands)	Specific muscle tests IM and acupuncture points IM and wrist pulses

BALANCING: CORRECTIONS AND TREATMENT

The aim of Kinesiology is to create a state of health and harmony by bringing all aspects of the person into balance. This is achieved by correcting any imbalances found in assessment, using a synthesis of energy-balancing techniques and corrections drawn from chiropractic, osteopathy, acupuncture and other healing disciplines. Some of the corrections are standard therapeutic techniques, while others are unique to Kinesiology. Individual Kinesiologists often add corrections of their own that are not part of Kinesiology.

One of the most remarkable and unique advantages of Kinesiology is the way in which it uses the body itself to determine what is needed. For example, once an imbalance has been identified through a weak muscle response, the practitioner can use that weak response to find out exactly what corrections or treatment that body needs to change the response from weak to strong. This relieves the practitioner of having to decide what is required, although of course he or she does have to know what options to offer. It also means that a system like Touch For Health, designed for laypersons, is safe to use.

A second unique advantage is the instantaneous feedback from the body about what it needs, without having to wait for days or weeks to find out whether a treatment is appropriate.

A third distinctive and very useful advantage is that muscle testing also gives both Kinesiologist and client immediate feedback as to whether the correction or treatment has worked. Immediately after carrying out the correction, the practitioner re-tests the formerly weak muscle. If it is now strong, this not only shows the practitioner that the correction has been effective: the client will feel the difference in the muscle response and will also know that it has worked. This knowledge produces a positive attitude, which in itself promotes the healing process. Anchoring the positive change in this way also allows the person's body to make the necessary internal adjustments to the change that has just taken place. And of course, it is a great deal speedier and more efficient than, for example, taking a medical drug for several days or weeks before knowing whether it helps or whether it has side-effects.

TYPES OF CORRECTION

Because of the diversity of Kinesiology it is not possible in this book to describe all the corrections and treatments given by the various systems and branches. The following are commonly used in AK, Touch For Health and the main branches of Kinesiology. When a muscle is found to be weak, any one or a combination of a number of standard corrections may strengthen it. Standard corrections are:

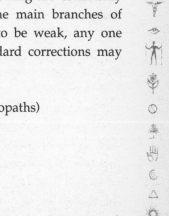

- Manipulation (chiropractors and osteopaths)
- Massaging neuro-lymphatic reflexes
- Holding neuro-vascular reflex points
- Meridian tracing
- Holding acupressure points
- Muscle reprogramming

Additional standard corrections are:

- Cross Crawl – Right-/left-brain integration
- Emotional Stress Release (ESR)
- Nutritional balancing

These are only a few of the most commonly used corrections; there are many more, some of which are described in Chapter 6.

MASSAGING NEURO-LYMPHATIC REFLEXES

Neuro-lymphatic reflexes are specific areas or points located on the front and back of the body, relating to the lymphatic system. They were first mapped out in the early part of the twentieth century by Frank Chapman, an osteopath (see Owens Charles, *An Endocrine Interpretation of Chapman's Reflexes*, American Academy of Osteopathy, USA, 1963). During his researches, George Goodheart found correlations between Chapman's reflexes and specific muscles.

The lymphatic system is one of the body's most important drainage systems, and its proper functioning is essential to good health. Stimulating the neuro-lymphatic reflexes by deep massage has the effect of stimulating the lymphatic system via the nervous system. For example, the neuro-lymphatic massage area for the colon (the large intestine) is found down the outside of the legs, from the hips to the knees; massaging this area can relieve constipation by stimulating the colon.

If the lymphatic system is sluggish in a particular area the relevant muscle will test weak; stimulating the appropriate reflex point has the effect of instantly strengthening the muscle concerned. Neuro-lymphatic reflexes are activated by deep pressure for about 25-30 seconds. While they are being massaged the person may feel some discomfort, but this diminishes quickly.

In the 1930s a Californian chiropractor, Dr Bennet, discovered areas on the head which, when lightly held, seemed to stimulate the blood supply to specific organs and glands; his discovery was aided by the use of a Fluoroscope, a kind of moving X-ray machine. Dr Goodheart discovered that holding these points, which he called neuro-vascular reflex points, could also restore strength to weak muscles; when weakness was due to poor circulation, again he discovered correlations between specific points and specific muscles.

These points are located mainly on the head, and are held lightly for one or two minutes, or longer, until a pulse (not directly connected with the heartbeat) can be felt and is steady. The bilateral points (points on bòth sides of the head) are held until the pulses synchronize.

The effect of holding these points is deep relaxation and there is no discomfort. For example, the neuro-vascular reflexes for the stomach are located on the brow, above the eyebrows. These are also emotional stress release reflexes. Holding these reflexes improves circulation to the stomach and reduces stress.

MERIDIAN TRACING

We have already established that specific muscles are connected energetically to specific meridians and organs and glands. This connection is used not only diagnostically in assessment, but also therapeutically in correction and treatment.

Meridians are energy pathways in the body through which *qi*, or life-energy, flows. In Kinesiology muscle testing, a weak muscle can indicate a restriction in the flow of energy in the meridian connected with that muscle.

The flow of energy can be stimulated by tracing the meridian pathway with the fingers in the appropriate direction, directly on the client's body or within 2 in/5 cm of it. During

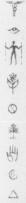

the tracing process both practitioner and client often feel sensations such as heat, cold or tingling (sensations which are quite common when subtle energy is being worked on or activated).

For example, the central meridian, which runs up the centre line of the body, finishing at the lower lip, interconnects with all the other meridians and with the brain. Stimulating the flow of energy in this meridian by tracing can increase the energy supply to the brain, enhancing brain function.

HOLDING ACUPRESSURE POINTS

As well as tracing meridians to stimulate the flow of energy, Kinesiology uses specific acupuncture points to stimulate or sedate the energy in meridians. This has a balancing effect on the muscles, organs or glands connected with that meridian.

The usual Kinesiology treatment consists of lightly holding two acupuncture points for a minute or two until their pulsations synchronize. During the process it sometimes happens that the person and/or the practitioner can feel an energy change, perhaps experiencing a rush of energy, or a feeling of lightness, heat or coolness.

MUSCLE REPROGRAMMING

Sometimes the correction required is not related to any of the systems already described, but lies in the muscle programme itself, that is in the messages transmitted between the muscle and the brain.

On occasions a muscle just needs to be 'wakened up'. Manually stimulating either end of the muscle (the origin and insertion – i.e. the end of the muscle attached to non-moving bone and the end attached to moving bone) for a few seconds is enough to 'switch on' the communication, so that the muscle will now test strong.

However, many chronic muscle problems can occur when a muscle 'switches off' or changes its programme in response to injury or trauma, in order to protect itself, and then fails to 'switch on' again and return to normal afterwards. This can cause the other muscles which work with it to malfunction as well.

A Kinesiologist can identify these patterns of muscle imbalance or malfunction and can reprogramme the muscles now that the danger is past. This is done by going to the belly (the centre) of the muscle and pulling apart its fibres (the spindle cells) for a few seconds. The technique is not painful. This sends a message to the brain that the fibres are too long, and the brain responds by contracting them, so that the previously weak muscle is now strong. The reverse process, pushing the fibres in the belly of the muscle together, enables tight muscles to relax. This second method can also be used to relieve cramp and muscle spasm.

CROSS CRAWL – RIGHT-/LEFT-BRAIN INTEGRATION

As explained in Chapter 4, the brain has two hemispheres, right and left, each controlling the opposite side of the body. Most people have one dominant hemisphere, usually the left, which is why the majority of the population is right-handed. However, we function at our best when both hemispheres are activated and working together as an integrated whole.

Cross Crawl, or re-patterning, was first developed in 1960 by Drs Doman and Delacato to help brain-damaged children. Since then it has been developed and is used in Kinesiology to improve the co-ordination of normal children and adults.

As a Kinesiology exercise, Cross Crawl is used both to test for and to enhance right-/left-brain hemisphere integration. It involves marching on the spot, lifting the knees high, and touching the knees in turn with the opposite elbows.

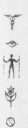

When there is an imbalance, the IM will test weak after the exercise has been performed. This can be corrected by getting the person to perform the same exercise for about a minute at a time, while looking in a direction which will change the IM from weak to strong; in right-handed people this usually means looking up to the left. This will assist the integration of the hemispheres. Other corrections for balancing brain activity include counting or humming while doing the Cross Crawl.

For more information, see the self-help techniques in Chapter 6, and the section on Educational Kinesiology in Chapter 7.

EMOTIONAL STRESS RELEASE (ESR)

To return to the Triad of Health, emotional balance is necessary for complete balance and harmony. Emotional stress can also be a primary factor in muscle imbalance, and can affect structure and body chemistry. ESR is a very simple yet powerful technique for helping people to deal with stress instantly and effectively.

George Goodheart discovered the emotional stress reflex by observing that people suffering from extreme stress or trauma showed visible reddened areas on the forehead, above the eyebrows. He found that if he held these reflexes lightly while the person mentally re-experienced the stress, the person's perception of the stress would change, and he or she would feel better able to deal with it.

Recent scientific research into the function of the brain, using CAT and functional MRI scans, shows that there are indeed emotional thinking circuits in the frontal cortex. The emotional stress release reflexes used in kinesiology are in the same location.[1]

[1] *New Scientist Supplement*, April 1996.

The Physiology of Stress

When the body/mind is under stress the blood supply is drawn away from the peripheral areas of the skull and directed to the large muscles of the body. In acute stress this is called the fight-or-flight mechanism. In this state, the front part of the brain performs less efficiently: this is the part of the brain we use when thinking without emotional attachment. At the same time, the more instinctive, back part of the brain, programmed by past memories and basic, primitive survival mechanisms reacts instantly to the stress by sending a chain of chemical messages through the body. The adrenal glands (which sit on top of the kidneys, at the back above the waist) send adrenalin into the bloodstream, which raises blood-sugar levels and increases the blood supply to the heart, legs and major muscles, to prepare the body for fighting the bear at the cave entrance, or running away from it. These days we very rarely have physically to fight or flee for our lives, but our brains and body chemistry still react to acute stress in this instinctive way.

Using Emotional Stress Release (ESR)

The good news is that we can do something about this, immediately and effectively through the ESR technique, which involves holding the ESR reflexes while the stressed person re-experiences in as much detail as possible the situation that is causing stress and all the emotions associated with it. This can also be used to clear emotional imbalances identified through the Five Elements. The ESR reflexes are also the neuro-vascular reflexes for the stomach. The stomach is not only the place where we digest our food; it is also where we digest our emotions – hence the sensation of 'butterflies in the stomach' induced by anxiety, and the fact that stomach ulcers are often stress-related.

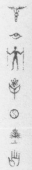

Holding the ESR reflexes very lightly encourages the blood supply to the stomach and the frontal lobes of the brain. This part of the brain does not react to past memory, but functions in present time, and is spontaneous, creative and objective.

Initially, while the person is re-experiencing the stress, no pulse is felt on these points. Gradually, after a minute or two, erratic pulses may be felt on both sides. Eventually, after anything from a few to 10 minutes, these pulses become synchronized and steady. When this happens there is a profound change in the person's physiology. The whole body relaxes, the breathing slows down and deepens, and the person no longer feels affected by the stressful situation.

The original cause of stress has not actually changed or disappeared; what has changed is the person's *perception* of the stress. Often during the stress release process new solutions emerge from the creative part of the brain, and the purely emotional response is replaced by a balanced one.

This is a wonderfully non-invasive method of offering help. The practitioner does not need to know what the person's problem is, nor does he or she need counselling skills to use it effectively. The technique can be used safely to deal with any kind of stress, from fear of flying to dealing with problems in the past, present or future. You can use it yourself to help friends in a crisis, and for self-help (see page 85).

Bach Flower Remedies

Bach Flower and other flower remedies are also often used in emotional balancing. These remedies are plant essences in homoeopathic form and relate to emotional states. Muscle testing can be used to select the most effective remedy needed to correct an emotional imbalance. A few drops are usually taken on the tongue every day, for as long as is required.

As well as developing their own methods of emotional assessment, all the branches of Kinesiology have developed their own corrections and treatments for emotional balancing. Some of these are described in Chapters 6 and 7.

NUTRITIONAL BALANCING

To return again to the Triad of Health, nutrition plays a very important part in our chemical balance. A nutritional imbalance can be a primary factor in structural imbalance, and can also affect the mind and the emotions.

As explained in Chapter 4, every muscle tested in Kinesiology has a nutritional factor, and muscle testing enables the Kinesiologist to give dietary recommendations to enhance the functioning of the body, chemically, structurally and mentally. To return to the example of the latissimus dorsi, which is related to the pancreas and blood-sugar levels: if it is weak for nutritional reasons, it will be strengthened by taking foods rich in Vitamin A, such as green, leafy vegetables, and by reducing sugar intake.

Some branches of Kinesiology, such as Clinical Kinesiology, Health Kinesiology and Biokinesiology, use their own individual methods of nutritional balancing and allergy correction.

OPTIONS FOR BALANCING

With all these choices for correction and treatment, when and how are they selected and applied, and where does the Kinesiologist start the balancing process?

Every muscle has associated neuro-lymphatic reflexes, neuro-vascular reflexes, a meridian and acupressure points; stimulating the appropriate points will strengthen a muscle which is weak due to under-energy. ESR and nutritional support can also strengthen a weak muscle, as can many other corrections and treatments not described here.

Here is an example of the corrections for one muscle and how these are selected. The same procedure is used for all muscles.

The pectoralis major clavicular muscle is located on both sides of the upper chest; it starts at the collar-bone and attaches to a bone in the front of the shoulder. It is associated with the stomach meridian and the stomach.

The neuro-lymphatic reflexes for this muscle are located on the front of the body just under the breast on the left side, on the back of the body between the shoulder blades (about half way down) and on either side of the spine.

The neuro-vascular reflexes are two points on the bumps of the brow (the ESR reflexes).

The stomach meridian starts under the eye and finishes on the second toe (next to the big toe). It runs along both sides of the body.

Acupressure holding points are located on the hands and feet.

The ESR reflexes are used for emotional corrections.

Nutritional support consists of foods rich in Vitamin B Complex (whole grain, brewer's yeast, etc.). Dietary recommendations are to avoid sugars and sweets, especially before meals.

The Kinesiologist, having found a weak pectoralis major clavicular muscle, asks the client to touch any of the points listed above, in order to find out which point or points will change the response from weak to strong. These are tested in the order listed above.

The Kinesiologist will then carry out the correction(s) indicated, and having done this will re-test the previously weak muscle to confirm that the correction has worked.

The Kinesiologist may go on to challenge the point, to find out whether the balancing for that muscle is complete or whether further corrections are necessary.

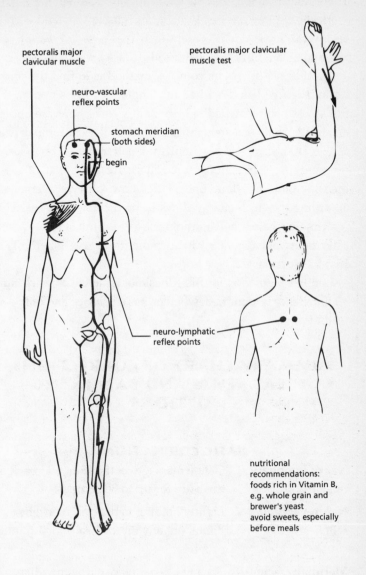

pectoralis major
clavicular muscle

neuro-vascular
reflex points

stomach meridian
(both sides)

begin

pectoralis major clavicular
muscle test

neuro-lymphatic
reflex points

nutritional
recommendations:
foods rich in Vitamin B,
e.g. whole grain and
brewer's yeast
avoid sweets, especially
before meals

Figure 4

There are a number of balancing options. The simplest is to work through a series of 14 or more muscle tests and correct each weak muscle as it is identified. This is called 'Fix as you go', and is taught in the TFH Level 1 (Basic) workshop.

Another, slightly more complex method is to find the priority imbalance(s) as described in Chapter 4. In this option, the full assessment is carried out before any corrections are undertaken. Kinesiologists using this method will record imbalances as they find them, and may look for a pattern based on theories of energy flow in acupuncture. There are a number of these theories (an important one is the Law of Five Elements), according to which energy flows in predictable patterns. This information helps the Kinesiologist to find the starting point. (The theory of energy flow in acupuncture is taught in the TFH Level 2 workshop.)

Another method is for the Kinesiologist to check, each time an imbalance is identified, whether it is a priority, and only correct it if it is.

SUMMARY CHART OF CORRECTIONS, TREATMENTS AND BALANCING OPTIONS

BASIC CORRECTIONS

Neuro-lymphatic reflexes	Gentle massage on the front and back of the body for up to 30 seconds
Neuro-vascular reflexes	Lightly holding neuro-vascular reflex points (mainly on the head) for 1 minute or more
Meridian tracing	Tracing the pathway of the meridian either on the body or within 2 in/5 cm of the body

| Acupressure holding points | Lightly holding two pairs of specific acupuncture points simultaneously for 1 minute |
| Muscle reprogramming | Origin and insertion (O & I):
  Gently activating both ends of the muscle
Spindle cell mechanism:
  Working on the fibres in the belly of the muscle, pulling apart to strengthen and pushing together to weaken for a few seconds |

ADDITIONAL CORRECTIONS

Cross Crawl	Cross Crawl exercise combined with specific eye movements and brain activity
Emotional Stress Release	Lightly holding points on each side of the brow till both pulses are steady and synchronized
Nutritional balancing	Balancing the whole person, and offering dietary recommendations

BALANCING OPTIONS

'Fix As You Go'	Correcting imbalances as they are identified
Priority balance	Completing assessment without corrections and finding the priority for balancing that will also correct other imbalances
Priority correction	Correcting only those imbalances that are a priority as they are identified
Energy patterns	Using the patterns of energy flow dictated by acupuncture theories and the Law of Five Elements

ADDITIONAL AND
SELF-HELP TECHNIQUES

This chapter draws on just some of the additional techniques used in AK, TFH and branches of Kinesiology. In each case a description is given of what is tested or assessed, the corrections used and how these can be used for self-balancing. You may find variations in the way these are used by different Kinesiologists. If you have not read the more technical Chapters 4 and 5, descriptions of some of the tests and corrections used for self-help are repeated here.

These self-help techniques are intended for use by people of all ages, including children, who are in good health; if you are suffering from a disease or illness, you should seek professional help before embarking on any self-help balancing.

Practising these techniques regularly can improve your health, performance and sense of well-being, and as they only take a few seconds or minutes to do they can easily be fitted into a busy schedule and practised on a daily basis. If you want to learn more about them you might like to attend a Touch For Health workshop. Details of training schools and organizations are given in Appendix B.

To give you an idea of the wide scope of Kinesiology, a number of techniques which cannot easily be used for self-balancing are also listed here, although they are not described in detail.

We all have a choice in life as to whether we drift with the tide and accept the consequences, or ask ourselves, 'What do I really want?' Setting ourselves clear goals gives us a sense of direction: one important result of defining a goal is that it immediately becomes much more attainable. This has applications in every area of life: relationships, health, work, and play. A good example is the story of Helen (page 157), whose life changed once she had defined a positive outcome for herself.

In the context of Kinesiology, goal-setting helps both the client and the practitioner to be clear about what they are working towards. In life generally, better results are achieved if they are related to a goal. The same applies in Kinesiology, when assessment, corrections and treatment are all linked to a goal, as opposed to being random.

Goal-setting methods are similar to those used in NLP (Neuro-Linguistic Programming), a system based on the study of how rather than what we think, and how we process sensory information. Some branches of Kinesiology have drawn on and adapted NLP theory and techniques.

NLP sets certain guidelines for setting goals and well-formed outcomes. For example, it is important to state goals in the positive: 'I want to enjoy the feeling of freedom and movement in my back,' rather than 'I don't want to have backache.' The moment you think of the state you desire, you start to have some sensory awareness of it; you begin to experience just what the positive outcome will be like, rather than being stuck with the idea of yourself in pain.

For goals to be successful, they need to be realistic and attainable. Muscle testing can be used to help you find the best goal for yourself, together with the emotions that are linked with it. The various branches of Kinesiology use a number of different methods for testing and setting goals.

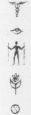

Get into the habit of setting goals for yourself. Start with small ones that you know are within your reach, and build up into bigger ones. You could begin each morning by setting a goal for the day. Keep your goal in mind; and be aware of any factors that might get in the way. These are dealt with in the next section.

GOAL-BALANCING

It is important to acknowledge that there are often hidden factors that conflict with our apparent desire for change. For example, a person with a back problem may be unconsciously benefiting by getting extra love and attention, or a woman with a weight problem may be protecting herself from male attention. Achieving goals often entails making changes which can confront us with new and possibly threatening challenges.

There are a number of ways of dealing with these factors when goal-setting in co-operation with a Kinesiologist. To begin with, once the goal has been set and the related emotions identified, the Kinesiologist can link all further assessment and corrections with the goal and balance the body/mind in relation to it.

Another method is to use muscle testing to identify hidden resistances. As has been explained, the left hemisphere of the brain (the 'logic' hemisphere in most people) controls the right side of the body, and the right hemisphere (in most people the more creative, intuitive side of the brain) controls the left side of the body. An indicator muscle (IM) on the right side of the body can be used to obtain a response from the logic hemisphere, and one on the left side to obtain the response from the creative, intuitive hemisphere. For a goal to be successful, both hemispheres must give a positive response. When there is a hidden conflict one hemisphere, often the left brain, may give a positive (i.e. strong IM) response to a statement of the goal, while the other hemisphere gives a negative (i.e. weak) response; it can also happen that both IMs are weak.

Brain Integration – Self-help

One correction for hidden conflict is 'brain integration', developed by Paul Dennison, Edu-K, which uses a physical metaphor for integrating the two hemispheres. This is what you do:

- Extend your arms horizontally to the sides, palms forward.
- Imagine that your left brain is in the left palm and your right brain in the right palm. (You may find this easier to do with your eyes closed.)
- Now, thinking about your goal, very slowly let your palms, still containing each hemisphere, come together so that they meet in the centre and your fingers interlock.
- Take a moment to sense the integration.

If you don't feel you have achieved full integration the first time, you can repeat this several times.

Goal Balancing: Stress Release – Self-help

If you are aware without testing that thinking about your goal is stressful for you, you can use the basic Emotional Stress Release technique (described on page 88).

PSYCHOLOGICAL REVERSAL

This is another way of dealing with the hidden conflicts that prevent people from realizing their goals. It was developed by Dr Roger Callahan.

When there is repeated failure to achieve a goal, this is sometimes due to what in Kinesiology is called 'psychological

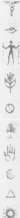

reversal'. This is shown when a strong IM weakens when the person states his or her positive goal, and strengthens when he or she thinks of not attaining it.

Although some counselling or further Kinesiology assessment may be required to find the cause, there is a very quick and simple correction for this. This consists of tapping an acupuncture point (called Small Intestine 3), which is located on the outside edge of the hand near the crease formed when you make a fist (see Figure 5a).

The Kinesiologist taps this point on both of the client's hands very rapidly, three times per second, for 20 seconds, while the client repeats: 'I have complete confidence in myself and accept myself as I am.' This changes the energy pattern in the meridian, which releases negativity. Re-testing will now confirm a positive or strong IM response to the positive goal.

Psychological Reversal – Self-help

- Think of a goal that you have been unable to attain. Be aware of how you feel.
- Tap the points as described above, or ask a friend to tap them, while you repeat the statement: 'I have complete confidence in myself and accept myself as I am.'
- Think of your goal again, and be aware of how you feel now.

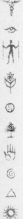

TEMPORAL TAP

This is a Kinesiology technique for embedding positive affirmations or goals, and consolidating positive change in the present. It can be used to enhance any changes you are making. It involves tapping with the fingers along the temporosphenoidal (TS) line on the skull, which forms a fan shape around and above the ears (see Figure 5b). This is the place where the

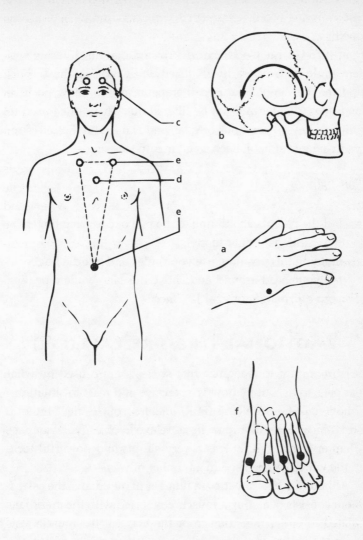

Figure 5: Self-help Reflex Points: a. psychological reversal;
b. temporal tapping; c. ESR; d. thymus tapping; e. polarity and
visual inhibition; f. gait (walking)

body/mind filters incoming sensory information so that we are not overwhelmed by too much information coming at us at any one time.

In 1975 George Goodheart discovered that this filtering system could be temporarily switched off by tapping the TS line, and that this could be used therapeutically to allow positive messages to enter and not be filtered out. This can be used to enhance any affirmations or goal, and is useful to help to support changes of habit such as giving up smoking.

Self-help

- Put the pad of each thumb to the pad of each ring finger (in the emotional finger mode).
- Holding this position, use your index and middle fingers to tap your head around and above the ears, while repeating your affirmation or goal 10 times.

EMOTIONAL STRESS RELEASE (ESR)

It is important to recognize that stress is not caused by what happens to us, but by how we perceive and react to situations. Emotional Stress Release (ESR) enables you to view hitherto stress-inducing situations in a relaxed, objective way (see Chapter 5, page 74. ESR is a very simple and powerful technique which can be used in a number of ways.

Although stress can affect a number of meridians, the assessment consists of testing a muscle connected with the meridians related to either the stomach or the brain. If the muscle tests strong at first but weakens when the person thinks of a stressful situation, then ESR is indicated.

Like other Kinesiology techniques, ESR is very helpful in dealing with all kinds of day-to-day stresses. Used in this way it is safe and brings balance and harmony. Sometimes hidden emotions come to the surface, and as they are released may give rise to tears of relief, which also frees held-in stress. However, anyone with a medical disorder such as clinical depression should seek professional help.

Although it is an advantage to have someone else holding the ESR points, you can use the technique on yourself with equal benefit, or offer to do it for another person.

Basic ESR – Self-help

The ESR points are two reflex points, located on the small bumps on your brow called *frontal eminences*; they are found halfway between the midline of your eyebrows and your hairline (see Figure 5c).

- Close your eyes and place your fingertips lightly over these points.
- Now think about the situation or issue that is troubling you. Experience it as fully as possible, by being aware of what and who you see, hear and feel, and even taste or smell.
- Keep re-running the scene through in your mind; after a while you will actually find it difficult to focus on it.
- When this happens, open your eyes, think again about the situation, and be aware of how you feel about it now.

This process can take anything from one to ten minutes. As you hold the points, you may feel pulsing, erratic at first. As the two pulses synchronize your stress is diffused.

ESR with a Friend

If you want to help a troubled friend you can offer to hold his or her ESR points while your friend processes stress. This can be done in silence; there is no need for him or her to share the

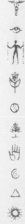

stressful experience with you. This is a respectful and caring way to give help to anyone who is emotionally upset.

ADVANCED ESR

Advanced ESR incorporates the emotional finger mode and eye rotations adapted from NLP by Dr Wayne Topping and used in Biokinesiology (see page 118). Holding the emotional finger mode activates the emotional centres in the brain, and when we move our eyes into different positions we access information from different parts of the brain, such as images and memories. For example, when we look up we are accessing the part of the brain where we visualize, or see pictures. Any stress triggered in this way by eye rotation can be released through the ESR technique.

Advanced ESR is interchangeable with standard ESR, and can be used at any time.

Advanced ESR – Self-help

- Bring together the pads of the thumbs and ring fingers of both hands.
- Now place the index and middle fingers of both hands on the ESR points on your brow.
- Think about the stressful situation or issue, and at the same time very slowly rotate your eyes, first in one direction and then in the other, first with your eyes closed and then with your eyes open. You may wish to repeat this.
- Now think of the stressful situation again. Notice how it seems to have changed.

ESR: PAST, PRESENT AND FUTURE

You are now familiar with the basic ESR technique. This can be applied to stresses from the past, the present, or anticipated in the future.

One way of changing your reaction to unhappy memories is to hold your ESR points while you recall the event in as much detail as possible. When you have done this, imagine how it could have been different and more positive. What did you need at that time? What didn't you know that you know now? Who (possibly including God, if this is your belief) could have helped you? What would you like to have done, or not to have done? Create a new version, incorporating all the resources you can think of that would have made it better for you. In doing this, you are creating another way of perceiving the stressful experience, and creating helpful inner resources for yourself.

You can now ask yourself if those resources could be useful in dealing with any present situation, or a similar problem in the future. Think of a similar situation that might cause you stress in the future, and construct it in your mind, including all the resources you now have for dealing with it. Test it out by making any changes in the scenario that would improve your performance. Repeat this several times.

You are now prepared to deal with this future event more effectively than you were before.

DEHYDRATION AND WATER

70 per cent of the human body consists of water. The kidneys, which are the blood's filtration system, can be affected by an inadequate water intake, and this will affect your general health. For example, there is an important muscle connected with the kidneys called the psoas which, when weak, can cause backache. The psoas will test weak if the body is dehydrated, and can strengthen the instant water is taken in.

Most of us do not drink enough water. Did you know that in the course of 24 hours we can lose the equivalent of 10 glasses

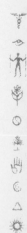

of water simply through breathing, sweating and excretion through the kidneys and intestines?

Dehydration first manifests in the tissues of the skin. The Kinesiology test for dehydration is to pull the skin of the scalp by gently tugging the hair, while testing an indicator muscle. If the IM weakens, this indicates a need for water.

Self-help

You do not need to be tested for dehydration to ensure that you drink enough water – 6–8 glasses a day. Pure spring or filtered water is better than tap water, which contains impurities and chlorine.

Like all Kinesiologists, osteopath Ashley Robinson stresses the importance of water. One of his patients used to get acute back problems two or three times a year. Although he recovered fairly quickly with treatment, he would have liked to avoid it in the first place. One day he visited Ashley for treatment on the day when the problem occurred (he usually had to wait a few days for an appointment). His psoas muscle was weak, and he weakened to the hair-tugging test, indicating dehydration. Following this he began drinking more water and less tea: his back problem has not recurred.

STIMULATING THE IMMUNE SYSTEM

THE THYMUS GLAND

The thymus gland plays an important role in the immune system, the body's defence system, and therefore in our ability to fight infections. So its healthy function is vital to our overall health. Stress affects the thymus, as can infections; in extreme cases it can shrink to half its normal size and weight in a period of 24 hours. This is one reason why we are more likely to get ill when we are very stressed.

The thymus is located in the middle of the upper chest, and is the gland associated with the heart (see Figure 5d); it actually seems to be affected by the amount of love a person gives and receives. This may explain why elderly people living alone, who have a heart condition, often experience an improvement when they acquire a domestic pet to look after and love.

Kinesiologists test the thymus by Therapy Localization (TL): the client touches the centre of the upper chest while the practitioner tests an IM. If the IM weakens, this can indicate that the gland is underactive.

Self-help

The healthy function of the thymus can be encouraged by simply tapping this area of the chest with all four fingers and the thumb of one hand, to a waltz rhythm for about 20 seconds. You can help to keep your body healthy by doing this every day.

IMPROVING VISION, HEARING AND CO-ORDINATION

VISUAL INHIBITION

Sometimes looking in a particular direction, or moving the eyes back and forth when reading, can cause stress. In Kinesiology this is called Visual Inhibition. It can relate to many problems, including poor co-ordination and dyslexia. A symptom of Visual Inhibition is unsteadiness or lack of balance when looking down as you go down stairs, or feeling tired when reading.

Kinesiologists assess this by testing an IM while the client keeps his or her head straight and looks up, then down, then to both sides. If the IM weakens when the client is looking in any of these directions, this indicates there is some stress caused by these eye positions.

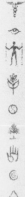

This is corrected by keeping the eyes in the position that weakened the IM and simultaneously massaging some acupuncture points. (This was one of the corrections that helped to improve Jimmy's vision in the case history in Chapter 2.) Educational Kinesiology uses many further tests for vision.

Self-help

You can help to keep your eyes stress-free by using the following techniques:

- Put one hand on your navel, and with the thumb and fingers of the other hand rub two points just beneath your collarbone, about 4 in/10 cm apart (see Figure 5e).
- At the same time, keeping your head straight, very slowly rotate your eyes all the way round one way, then all the way back the other way.
- This takes only about 30 seconds, can be done at any time, and can be repeated several times a day if you wish. Watch for the improvement.
- You can also practise an exercise called 'Lazy 8'. Imagine (or draw) a large figure 8 lying on its side. Keeping your head still, follow the outline of the 8 with your eyes, starting in the direction of the upwards left-hand curve. You can do this several times.

HEARING AND BALANCE

As well as their obvious function in hearing, our ears are important in other ways: the inner ear affects our balance, and the outer ear contains a map of the whole body. (A branch of acupuncture, auricular acupuncture, treats points on the ears to affect all parts of the body.)

Our ears also emit energy and draw it into the body. You may be able to feel this for yourself by placing each hand within

2 in/5 cm of your ears and slowly moving your hands up and then down. This energy can be assessed in Kinesiology by testing an IM while the person turns his or her head as far as possible to one side and then to the other. This activates neck muscles which affect the ears. If the IM weakens with either head turn, this indicates some imbalance in the ear energy. The Kinesiologist can correct it by getting the person to turn his or her head in the direction that weakened the IM, while firmly (but not painfully) pulling the ears, as if to unfold them, away from the ear-hole and working down from the top to the lobe.

This correction was used on an elderly gentleman whose hearing had been impaired during the Second World War, and led to a distinct improvement in his hearing.

Self-help

If you want to energize your ears, and thereby your whole body, firmly unfold your ears as described above. It should take about 15 seconds. This can also improve your balance, and has been found helpful in some cases of travel sickness.

CROSS CRAWL

Cross Crawl has already been described in Chapter 5. This exercise involves marching on the spot, swinging your arms and lifting your knees. As you do this, let each elbow touch the opposite knee in turn.

Cross Crawl is used both to test for and to improve integration between the two brain hemispheres. As a test, if a strong IM weakens after completing a few Cross Crawl movements (around 10), this indicates that there is stress, and a need for further integration. Educational Kinesiology (Edu-K) specializes in dealing with this kind of imbalance, and provides a range of tests to find the specific corrections required by each individual.

Practising Cross Crawl helps the logical, analytical hemisphere and the creative, intuitive hemisphere to work well together. Because each hemisphere controls the opposite side of the body, good integration between the two also means good bodily co-ordination. It is a helpful exercise for people with dyslexia and poor co-ordination, such as the little girl described in Chapter 7, who was clumsy and forgetful (see page 113).

The self-help correction described below is a general correction which has been beneficial to many people. If, however, you don't feel at ease doing it, stop, and consider consulting a practitioner in a one-to-one session.

Cross Crawl – Self-help

To improve your hemisphere balance and overall co-ordination, this is what you do:

- March slowly on the spot, as described above, for about 20 seconds.
- Once you can do this, repeat the exercise and at the same time slowly rotate your eyes first in one direction and then the other, or in a figure of eight lying on its side.

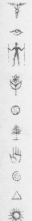

POLARITY SWITCHING

Like batteries, our bodies contain positive south-pole and negative north-pole polarities; as with batteries, these polarities affect our electrical circuits. Stresses of all kinds – mental, physical and chemical – can disturb our polarities, causing faulty signals in our electrical circuits, which in turn create confusion in our body and mind.

Each hand has a different dominant polarity. The left hand is north-pole and negative, the right hand south-pole and positive. The Kinesiology test for polarity switching is as follows:

The Kinesiologist tests an IM on both sides of the body. He or she then tests each IM individually, first with one hand, then with the other, and then with the first hand again, all in quick succession.

If the person's polarities are well-balanced, neither of the IMs will weaken when subjected to this rapidly repeated change in polarity from the testor's hand. However, if one does weaken, this indicates a disturbance in the person's polarities.

This imbalance is corrected by either the Kinesiologist or the client activating three sets of acupuncture points for about 10 seconds each, as follows:

Polarity Switching – Self-help

- Put one hand on your navel, and simultaneously massage the points just below your collar-bone and 4 in/10 cm apart (the same points as used for the eyes – see Figure 5e).
- Still with one hand on your navel, activate the points on your upper and lower lips by rubbing them.
- Finally, activate the point on your coccyx, at the base of your spine with one hand on your navel.

If you want to keep your polarities well-balanced and to be able to think even more clearly than you already do, you can use this correction on yourself, and can repeat it several times a day.

GAIT (WALKING) MECHANISM

Sometimes tiredness when walking is caused by poor coordination of the muscles involved in moving the arms and legs. This is assessed by first testing these muscles individually to check that they are strong, then testing two muscles in combination: for example, simultaneously testing the left arm and the right leg raised forward in a walking position.

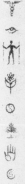

If any of these muscles test strong individually but weaken when tested in combination with another muscle, this shows a disturbance in the gait mechanism. Each combination of muscles has its corresponding set of correction points, which are found on the feet.

Self-help

If you want to keep all these muscles well co-ordinated, massage the points on your feet, near your toes, between the bones and on the sides of the big toe joint. Spend about 30 seconds on each foot. (See Figure 5f.)

SUMMARY CHART OF SELF-HELP TECHNIQUES

Goal-setting	Start each morning by setting a goal for the day. Make it realistic and attainable. Be aware of anything that stops you.
Goal-balancing brain integration	Extend your arms to the sides horizontally, palms forward. Imagine your left brain is in your left palm and your right brain in your right. Think about your goal and slowly bring both palms together till the fingers interlock.
Psychological reversal	Think of the goal you have been unable to attain. Tap a point on the side of each hand vigorously, saying 'I have complete confidence in myself and accept myself as I am.'
Temporal tap	Hold the pad of the thumb to the pad of the ring finger on both hands. Use your index and middle fingers to tap around and above

the ears, while repeating to yourself your affirmation or goal.

Emotional Stress Release (Basic ESR)	Lightly hold the ESR points (the bumps on your forehead). Re-experience your stress in detail, seeing, hearing and feeling it. Do this for 1–10 minutes.
Advanced ESR	Think about your stress. Hold your ESR points and slowly rotate your eyes first clockwise and then anti-clockwise.
ESR Past, Present and Future	Use the technique above, remembering the past cause of stress. Recreate it with all the resources you needed. Bring these into thinking of present or future events.
Water and dehydration	Drink 6–8 glasses daily of pure mineral or filtered water daily.
Thymus gland balancing	Tap the area of your chest over this gland (under the upper breastbone in the centre of the chest) for about 20 seconds, with all five fingers of one hand.
Eyes and vision	1. Place one hand on your navel. With the fingers and thumb of the other hold two points just under the collarbone, about 4 in/10 cm apart. Slowly rotate your eyes one way, then the other for 20 seconds. 2. Keeping your head still, follow with your eyes a large figure 8 on its side.
Ear balancing	Firmly unfold both ears, pulling outwards and working from the top down.
Cross Crawl	Marching slowly on the spot, bring each elbow to touch the opposite raised knee. At

the same time slowly rotate your eyes one way, then the other, and in a figure of eight on its side for a total of 20 seconds.

Polarity switching

Holding your navel, simultaneously massage the following acupuncture points for 10 seconds each:

1. 2 points below the collarbone, 4 in/10cm apart
2. points on the upper and lower lips
3. the tip of the base of your spine

Gait (walking) balancing

Massage points on your feet near your toes, and in between the bones and on the side of the big toe joint; 30 seconds on each foot.

ADDITIONAL TECHNIQUES
(NON-SELF-HELP)

Not all Kinesiology corrections can be used for self-help or self-balancing; there are also some self-help techniques that require more detailed instructions than can be given here. There are, in fact, so many factors that can be assessed and corrected in Kinesiology that it is impossible to include them all in this book.

To give you an idea of the wider scope of Kinesiology, here are just some of the factors that can be assessed and corrected, which have not been described so far:

- *Pain and pain control*: Pain can be relieved instantly via the acupuncture system.
- *Old scar tissue*: A scar can break the flow of energy and weaken a meridian running through it. Massage and other treatments can correct this.

- *Chakra imbalance*: The chakra are centres of energy found in the energy field and in the body. Kinesiology can test for imbalances in the chakra, and uses a range of healing techniques to balance them.
- *Blood-pressure*: A simple test, not involving machines, can be used to check whether your blood-pressure is balanced for you. If not, special polarity balancing can often help to correct it. This should also be monitored by BP readings.
- *Breathing*: Faulty breathing can affect your health. Kinesiology can improve the function of the muscles involved.
- *Phobia cure*: This technique is taken from *Five Minute Phobia Cure* by Dr R. Callahan. The theory is that the excessive emotional stress caused by a phobic reaction creates a temporary overenergy in one of the meridians, usually the stomach. Tapping the beginning or end of the meridian affected, while the person re-experiences the phobic state, re-balances the meridian. As a result, the phobic reaction disappears.
- *Accident trauma*: Our body cells and tissues, as well as our brains, hold memories. Sometimes, when someone undergoes a physical trauma such as an accident or a fall, the body attempts to protect itself by switching off certain muscles. Later, even though the person may not have a conscious memory of the event, his or her body retains the memory of the shock that occurred while it was in that particular position, and will weaken every time it is in that position.

  The Kinesiologist can clear this by putting the person's body in the position in which it was originally shocked, at the same time holding the ESR points. Sometimes this requires setting the scene in one's imagination and role-playing the accident.

• *Tibetan Figure-of-Eight Energy*: One of the patterns of energy flow that surrounds our body is the figure eight. This pattern occurs all over the body. Kinesiology can identify imbalances in this energy and can correct it by moving the energy in the energy field by hand in the appropriate direction.

BRANCHES OF KINESIOLOGY

Since the inception of Applied Kinesiology in 1964 and the subsequent development of Touch For Health in the early 1970s, a variety of branches of Kinesiology have evolved. More are developing all the time, but those described in this chapter are taught world-wide.

Before going on to describe the main branches, it is important to distinguish between systems and branches. We have defined Applied Kinesiology (AK) and Touch For Health (TFH) as systems, since they are the original systems, or models, from which all the branches have evolved. They are described in Chapter 1.

AK (and also CK, Clinical Kinesiology – see page 125) offers training only to already highly-trained professionals, while TFH offers basic Kinesiology training to everyone. TFH and trainings based on TFH such as FKP are pre-requisites for some, but not all, branches.

All the branches described here have been developed by people who, having trained in TFH and/or AK, have gone on to combine aspects of these systems with specialist knowledge and skills of their own. The majority of practitioners within these branches have also trained in TFH. The International Association for Specialist Kinesiologists, I-ASK, is an umbrella organization for professional kinesiologists practising specialized branches of kinesiology. It has standards for membership and has chapters (branches) throughout the world each of which has a register of members. See Appendix B for details of the I-ASK central office.

Training in all branches except AK and CK is open to anyone, including health practitioners and interested laypersons. Contact addresses for the branches described below are given in Appendix B.

All branches share the philosophy of health enhancement, and use muscle testing and some of the assessment and correction procedures of TFH/AK. All branches have as an ultimate goal the concept of the Triad of Health, that is, the balance of the structural, chemical and mental/emotional aspects of the human being. So what makes one branch different from another?

While there are many overlapping areas between them, what varies is the starting point and the route taken to reach the goal of balance and harmony. In Touch For Health, the initial focus of assessment is the muscle-meridian/organ-gland energy, and TFH corrections focus on energy balancing. By contrast, in Educational Kinesiology (Edu-K), for example, the initial focus of assessment is the electrical circuitry of the body/mind system, and the correction techniques differ in some respects from those of TFH, with additional corrections specific to Edu-K. On page 132 you will find a Summary Chart showing the chief differences between the main branches, and this chapter includes descriptions of these branches together with case histories illustrating how they work in practice.

These case histories have been selected to demonstrate the wide range of problems to which Kinesiology can be applied. The fact that more case histories are included for some branches than for others does not mean that the branch concerned is either bigger or more successful than the others.

While these case histories include some instances of remarkable results, it would be wrong to give the impression that Kinesiology can cure everything. This is not the case. No practitioner heals another person: the body is constantly trying to heal itself, and Kinesiology aids and supports that process. Kinesiology grants the practitioner permission to work with a client, using the body's own wisdom to discover what is out of balance and what it needs for balance to be restored.

Muscle testing also gives both client and practitioner positive feedback which confirms that the healing process is going on. This knowledge, which is more than belief or faith, is a key factor in successful healing. However, the very fact that this biofeedback is so instantaneous can occasionally mislead people into imagining that Kinesiology is some kind of 'magic wand'. It is true that results can at times be rapid, but it is more usual for the healing process to be an ongoing one, which may take weeks or months to be completed.

FOUNDATION KINESIOLOGY PRACTITIONER (FKP) (TFH FOR PRACTITIONERS)

Strictly speaking, this training is an expansion of the existing parent system, TFH, rather than a branch. I developed this training in response to the demand from an increasing number of health professionals wanting to train in Kinesiology. These people wanted a more professional foundation training than that offered by TFH (which is designed for lay people) but were not eligible to do AK training. Some lay people who are not health professionals but want to train to be professional Kinesiologists also choose this training.

The FKP training is a structured course in two parts. It is taught over 14 days, usually over a period of seven months,

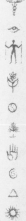

and includes home study and assessment. It teaches TFH in more depth with an emphasis on understanding the concepts underlying the TFH material. It allows more time to assimilate and consolidate the information and to develop competence in practical work.

The FKP training course offers an alternative to the TFH workshops and meets the changing needs in professional training and standards required by many countries today. For details of the content of TFH and FKP, see Appendix A.

PROFESSIONAL KINESIOLOGY PRACTITIONER (PKP)

The PKP workshops grew out of the increasing need for a programme that would enable Touch For Health students to expand on the AK foundations gained in their basic training.

In the mid-1980s the TFH Foundation's Faculty Head, Dr Bruce Dewe, along with his wife Joan, pioneered a new workshop series called Touch For Health 4 and 5. Dr Dewe, a medical doctor and long-standing member of ICAK, took from the parent system the essential procedures that had not been covered in John Thie's original work, those that did not require manipulative skills or medical training. With the benefit of his own clinical experience he made these procedures accessible to the large number of TFH graduates who were seeking professional training.

PKP is taught over four five-day workshops. It is a synthesis of the most useful and established AK procedures and the innovations from the non-manipulative Kinesiology field that have developed from the original Touch For Health classes. Most of the procedures and techniques now taught have in fact been researched and developed not only by Dr Dewe but also by the growing number of specialized Kinesiologists working with this system in clinical practice. Annual research evaluation workshops are held for graduates to assess new applications and to share their own findings.

This work initially became known as the Professional Health Provider, and more recently as the Professional Kinesiology Practitioner programme, an acknowledgement that Dr Thie's original vision of training laypersons in these skills had indeed given birth to an essentially new health professional.

As well as the clear, de-jargonized dissemination of complex information, the programme's uniqueness lies in its combination of a finger-mode system of identifying the most effective procedures for a client, with the underlying principle of identifying and bringing awareness to emotional factors at each stage of the balance.

The finger modes were originally discovered by an osteopath and Applied Kinesiologist, Dr Alan Beardall, founder of Clinical Kinesiology (see page 125). They give the practitioner access to information about which aspect – emotional, physical, biochemical, or electrical – is primarily in need of attention. Dr Beardall's original four basic modes (accessed simply by holding the thumb to the tip of each finger in turn) proved to be remarkably consistent, and have been adopted throughout the Kinesiology world.

The research by the Dewes and their colleagues has developed this seemingly universal body language into a highly accessible 'database' for the operator of what Beardall called the 'biocomputer'. This system has continued to grow; and the Dewes' system has brought it into more and more widespread use, since they recognized that people could be trained to a highly proficient standard without reference to PKP's parent system, AK.

The PKP programme is now, along with Edu-K (page 109) and the Three-in-One series (page 113) one of the most

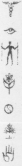

successful of the advanced courses available to the student of non-manipulative, holistic Kinesiology, and the one most directly concerned with the training of professional practitioners in a broad Kinesiology discipline. It is taught and practised in four of the five continents of the world.

The following case history includes treatment of hiatus hernia, a painful condition in which the stomach or oesophagus is squeezed out of its proper position, preventing food from being processed correctly and causing heartburn. The usual medical treatment is to prescribe medication to ease the heartburn, without dealing with the cause. Kinesiology provides a procedure which helps to balance the muscles around the diaphragm, allowing the stomach to return to its proper position; there are also some self-corrections which the Kinesiologist will suggest if appropriate.

CHRONIC EXHAUSTION

Julie, in her late thirties, was suffering from chronic exhaustion and severe aching of the muscles. PHP testing showed a tendency to hiatal hernia, a low level of thymus activity (the thymus plays an important part in the immune system) and the possibility of a Candida Albicans overgrowth (the fungal yeast infection often associated with Chronic Fatigue Syndrome, or M.E.). Her adrenal glands were also showing high levels of stress. In addition there were imbalances at the subtle energy levels, with the solar plexus centre appearing as priority. In the field of energy medicine, the solar plexus relates to a person's sense of personal power and responsibility.

Julie had been married at 17, and had lost a child through cot death. Several other relationships had turned out unhappily, and her son had been taken into care at the age of three.

Julie had spent most of her life trying to please her mother. As a result, she had become emotionally disempowered to the point where her solar plexus, her power centre, was too weak to sustain the proper functioning of her body in that area, resulting in the disturbances in adrenal and small intestine activity.

Julie had treatment at fortnightly intervals for three months. By working through the various procedures as indicated by the finger modes, while also identifying emotional factors and bringing Julie's awareness to those areas, she achieved previously unexperienced levels of energy and vitality. She celebrated by taking a holiday in Greece and joining a part-time massage course. Her aches had gone, her digestion was enormously improved, but the most marked change was the sparkle in her eye and the spring in her step.

From information supplied by Adrian Voce

This treatment was particularly interesting as it included elements on all levels. The correction for hiatus hernia is a very physical one, whereas balancing the solar plexus centre involves the subtle energies. The real shift in energy, however, came from enabling Julie to re-experience and heal some old traumas and, in particular, through altering her pattern of beliefs about herself. Her major breakthrough came when she allowed herself the right to say what she wanted to say, which was especially challenging for her in relation to her mother.

EDUCATIONAL KINESIOLOGY (EDU-K)

Educational Kinesiology, also known as Edu-K, has a wide range of applications, but is chiefly used for improving learning skills including reading, writing, numeracy, concentration, memory, etc. The simplest versions can be practised by children; it can also improve the all-round functioning of adults, since we all find ourselves at times in situations that demand clearer thinking, or that trigger learning problems.

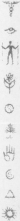

Edu-K was created by Dr Paul Dennison, Ph.D., in 1980. After working for 20 years at a remedial learning centre for children in California, he started to work closely with a chiropractor/Kinesiologist, and in 1979 trained in TFH. In 1982 he developed the Laterality Repatterning Programme (described below), and extended his work to include adults as well as children. Edu-K continued to develop as a study of the communications between the body and the brain, first focusing on the right and left hemispheres and then on other dimensions of the brain.

The Edu-K Foundation, based in the USA, offers training courses worldwide. These have been of interest to many practitioners and, in particular, to professional educationalists. Some Edu-K assessment and correction procedures have been incorporated into AK, TFH and other branches of Kinesiology.

HOW EDU-K WORKS

Educational Kinesiology uses muscle testing to identify stresses and imbalances that are caused by certain activities and movements which can affect co-ordination and performance in many areas. These are often the result of electrical disturbances which cause poor or faulty signals between the brain and the body. Imbalances can be caused by eye movements and head positions; it is not generally known, for instance, that for some people under stress, simply looking downwards will weaken all their systems. This not only affects people's gait – leading to unsteadiness when walking down steps – but, very importantly, can impair a child's ability to read, since reading almost always involves looking down.

While the simplest versions of Edu-K, such as the Brain Gym (see below) can be practised by schoolchildren in classrooms, the more advanced levels, such as Goal-balancing, are suitable to be taught only by trained practitioners in one-to-one situations. People trained in other areas, such as education or counselling, can achieve good results by adding Edu-K to their skills. Edu-K corrections include Laterality Repatterning, the Brain Gym, and Goal-setting.

Laterality Repatterning

This balances the left- and right-brain hemispheres. The Cross Crawl was originally devised in the 1960s by Drs Doman and Delacato, who used it very successfully to help brain-damaged children. Touching the hands to the opposite knees in Cross Crawl forces the left- and right-brain hemispheres to work simultaneously, and once the two hemispheres have 'learned' to work together communication between them is increased across the corpus callosum, the 'bridge' in the brain which connects the two halves. However, this technique alone is not enough for children or adults with learning or thinking difficulties, or dyslexia.

Dr Dennison observed that a more profound change came about when the person performing the Cross Crawl simultaneously activated their 'Gestalt' (i.e. holistic, non-logical) brain hemisphere by humming and turning the eyes in a specific direction. With another short procedure, and an intention to integrate, Repatterning can help everybody to be more efficient in new or difficult contexts. Thinking and behaviour become smoother and less stressful because the attention is better distributed.

The Brain Gym

This is a series of movements designed to bring about states of relaxed alertness for peak performance. Some re-distribute energy, some rebalance the left and right hemispheres, and others allow the supply of blood and oxygen, which is 'switched off' at times of stress, to flow back to the frontal cortex.

Goal-setting

When people start to expand out of their 'comfort zones ' into new areas, they may need help to make new neurological connections, which enables them to perform new tasks with less stress. Edu-K techniques help people to set themselves appropriate goals which are positive, active, clear and energizing.

The following examples show how Edu-K can benefit children, with or without specific learning difficulties.

A GROUP STUDY IN A LONDON SCHOOL

In October 1989 educationalist and Kinesiologist Vivienne Gill, with a colleague, introduced Edu-K to three classes of 9–10-year-olds in an inner-city school. They divided two of the classes so that they could compare the effects of using Edu-K techniques on 'experimental' and 'control' groups. The third class received Repatterning and Brain Gym exercises throughout.

By the following July, 1990, the overall results showed definite, measurable improvements in reading ability as a result of practising AK techniques, particularly in the class which had received the techniques throughout, and the children's ability to listen and get on with each other also improved.

Some children in particular benefited not only from improved reading ability, but also from increased self-confidence and self-esteem. One shy little girl, whose reading age soared from 6.11 to 9.11 years, said that she had lost her anxiety about reading, which she now really enjoyed.

One boy had been rather lonely, difficult and attention-seeking at the start. Between October 1989 and July 1991, a year after the first results were measured, his reading age went up from 7.8 to 13.6 years. Later he commented that he didn't notice any difference in himself, yet when reminded of how he had been two years earlier, he said, 'Oh, yes, I remember now. I didn't use to give a monkey's about anything, but now I think about life. I don't want to go on the dole when I grow up, I want a good job.'

A CHILD WITH POOR CO-ORDINATION

A girl of twelve who had been clumsy and forgetful for most of her life was brought to see a Kinesiologist by her mother. When she was assessed she was found to have poor integration between the right and left hemispheres, and although her dominant hemisphere was the non-logical, right hemisphere, she was also right-handed. This explained her poor co-ordination and her lack of ability to think logically, which caused forgetfulness. Edu-K balancing using Laterality Repatterning and other Edu-K techniques corrected this.

After three sessions the girl was in her school games team, and was generally better organized and less forgetful, though her parents took a while to notice that they no longer had to nag her continually about forgetting things. Her improvement was maintained, and at the end of that school year she won the effort prize for her class.

From information supplied by Kay McCarroll, MC,
MIPC, DHP and Vivienne Gill, M. Litt.

THREE-IN-ONE CONCEPTS

This unique approach to stress management has been developed since 1972 by Gordon Stokes, Training Director for the Touch For Health Foundation, and by Daniel Whiteside, who co-founded Three-in-One Concepts. Originally called 'One Brain', the training they developed was expanded to include other courses which combine elements of holistic health, body-energy work, neuro-science and original research. Three-in-One Concepts uses muscle testing to identify stresses,

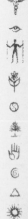

together with some corrections and treatments from AK and Touch For Health. The training consists of nine consecutive workshops and additional training.

The name reflects the expansion of the left/right hemisphere theory of brain function to include the integration of the front and back brain. When a person experiences emotional stress, the full capacity of the brain is not utilized; when the emotional stress is relieved, the brain is able to perceive and function in a calm, effective manner, with full access to left-brain logic and right-brain creativity. The whole brain operates as an integrated unit.

THE THREE-IN-ONE APPROACH

The first step is to identify the unresolved emotional stress and negative beliefs that prevent people from functioning at their full potential. The main method of assessment is to use an indicator muscle to identify priority stresses and corrections. Muscle testing is also used to assess at what level the stress is experienced – consciously, or subconsciously.

The corrections are selected from a broad spectrum of Stress-Defusion techniques, which are aimed at gently releasing negativity from the mind and body. If appropriate, follow-up exercises are assigned for the client to do at home.

TECHNIQUES TO HEAL THE PAST

Many present emotional, physical and behavioural problems have their roots in past traumas. Three-in-One techniques focus on clearing these, to restore our ability to make choices without the inhibiting consequences of our past experiences.

The Behavioural Barometer

This is a tool which helps the Kinesiologist to identify emotions the client may not be aware of: it consists of a systemized map of the emotions, including anger, fear, guilt and so on. The practitioner uses an indicator muscle to identify the primary upsetting emotion.

Age Recession

Age recession is a Three-in-One technique (also used in other branches of Kinesiology) to find out at what age a problem started. Using an indicator muscle the Kinesiologist asks whether a problem started at a particular age (between 20–15, 15–10, 10–5, and so on), and the muscle response will identify the period; the process is then continued in more detail to pinpoint the exact age when an original trauma took place.

The theory behind this is that although the person being tested may not have a conscious memory of, say, a trauma at the age of six months, the body/mind system holds the memory of the event, and it can be accessed as if it were happening in the present. The practitioner immediately uses Stress-Defusion techniques to heal the trauma, again as if it were happening in the present moment.

Three-in-One Defusion

This includes a wide choice of techniques, among them a version of Emotional Stress Release, in which the practitioner holds one hand on the stress release points on the forehead while the other hand holds the occiput, the back of the head, where the brain stores memories.

This can be carried out in silence; it is not necessary for the practitioner to know what the original trauma was, though on some occasions it may be appropriate for the practitioner and client to talk about what is going on. If the past experience was frightening, the client can re-experience it in a more detached way, as if watching a film, and can then have the opportunity to 're-write' the script and re-create the event as he or she

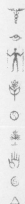

would have liked it to happen. While this is going on the Kinesiologist will continue to hold the Stress Defusion points.

The following story shows how healing past traumas can bring about important changes in the present, and how – as also recognized in Educational Kinesiology – learning difficulties often have their roots in emotional difficulties.

LEARNING DIFFICULTIES AND THE EMOTIONS

A man of 31 visited a One Brain practitioner. He told her that he was dyslexic, and had always had difficulty with reading, figures, and writing; he was about to start a new job, and was suffering from nervousness, lack of confidence and difficulty concentrating. His shoulders were bowed, his head drooped, and he told the practitioner that he suffered frequent nightmares about his school-days.

It emerged that when he was eight years old his school-teacher had thrown him against a wall and left him there. This event, followed by further reinforcement of his problems, had given rise to all his subsequent difficulties and lack of confidence.

He had six hour-long treatments over a period of three months, during which the practitioner treated him with One Brain techniques. His stress and lack of confidence began to disappear, and by the end of his treatments he was confident, was working happily in a new job, and had no more nightmares.

Sometimes problems are caused by traumas before birth, as in the case of a four-year-old who was unable to speak; age recession showed that he had been affected in the womb, when his mother had had to have an abdominal operation. After six months of Stress Defusions he was speaking clearly, and working happily at school. When children are treated in good time, results can happen remarkably quickly.

A boy of nine was taken to a practitioner because of dyslexia and bedwetting; his behaviour was also angry, though the anger appeared to be due more to frustration than to his natural temperament. The practitioner discovered that he was frightened of his father, and used One Brain Defusions to dissipate his fear.

At the end of one half-hour treatment, the little boy's anger and frustration had gone. The improvement continued, and over time he became happier and dry at night, while his schoolwork improved greatly. Perhaps even more importantly, his relationship with his father also improved considerably.

Another Three-in-One practitioner used age recession to help a mother with a problem child, in a rather unusual way.

MOTHER-CHILD BONDING

A woman who already had four children was having great difficulties with her youngest. At 3½ he was, in her words, 'hunted and haunted', had numerous tantrums, didn't want to be with her or without her, and wouldn't allow her to cuddle him.

The mother had had an unpleasant experience at his birth. She had wanted to give birth on all fours, feeling that this would be most comfortable for herself and the baby. The hospital staff disapproved, and although they allowed her to give birth as she wanted, they whisked the baby away as soon as he was born, so that she was unable to cuddle him until a few hours later.

The whole family came to the practitioner's house, and the little boy remained in another room playing with his brothers and sisters while the mother acted as a surrogate for him. This is very unusual: in accepted Kinesiology practice the surrogate always touches the patient. However, it was effective, no doubt because of the strong connection that exists between a mother and her child.

With the mother acting as surrogate, the child was regressed to the moment of birth. After a considerable amount of stress had been defused, he was brought in and asked if he would like to give his mummy a cuddle. The child immediately said, 'Yes,' and was lifted onto his mother's tummy, as if he had just been born.

Mother and child lay there, looking at each other and cuddling while the practitioner held the Stress-Defusion points a little longer. The practitioner commented afterwards that this moment was very moving. The bonding was complete.

The mother later wrote an account of the subsequent changes in the child: he now woke up happy instead of grizzling, no longer cried and screamed when she was out of sight, or threw tantrums if a brother or sister tried to share his toys. He started to ask questions and took an active interest in his surroundings and in books, which he had never looked at before. He had quiet, relaxed cuddles with his mother, and 'his eyes stopped being large, haunted saucers and became very beautiful, as if he were smiling to himself.'

From information supplied by Jeremy Glyn,
Janet Bradley and Daphne Clarke

Three-in-One work has helped people with a variety of stress-related problems including phobias (such as fear of heights and flying), M.E./Chronic Fatigue Syndrome, panic attacks and even alcoholism, as well as learning difficulties.

BIOKINESIOLOGY (BK)

Biokinesiology works on the connections between the internal organs and glands and positive and negative emotions. The Biokinesiology Institute was founded in 1972 by John Barton, a former computer designer with a deep interest in holistic therapies. He, his wife Margaret and their students produced a vast amount of research for early BK publications. Dr Wayne Topping, Ph.D., LMT, studied extensively with Barton, learning TFH and integrating some AK/TFH techniques with the BK approach. Using muscle testing, Therapy Localizing and Challenging, correlations were discovered between all parts of the body and positive and negative emotions.

Wayne Topping also added a new dimension to the Emotional Stress Release technique. This was the therapeutic application of eye positions drawn from NLP, which correlates specific eye positions with specific internal processes, such as visualizing the past or future, hearing, feeling, etc. Balancing is achieved by a combination of positive affirmations and Dr Topping's stress-release technique.

Wayne Topping has developed a series of workshops in BK.

CHRONIC PAIN-RELIEF

Diane, after a serious car accident six months before, was still suffering great pain in her neck, shoulders, arms, thighs and knees. Medical treatment had included wearing a collar and taking many painkilling drugs, with no benefit. Now she had been told that nothing more could be done medically, and that she would 'have to live with the pain'.

Diane was given a basic TFH balance of 14 muscles, followed by balancing the relevant muscles in the areas of pain. Certain meridians and reactive muscles were also corrected, but the pain persisted.

The practitioner next used Dr Topping's Stress Release work, while Diane re-experienced the accident; after this, all her muscles re-tested weak. She was then asked to rotate her eyes to the left and to the right; when her eye positions activated the brain at certain points, Diane reported that she felt pain in specific areas – the arms, elbow, shoulders, neck and legs.

Next the Emotional Stress Release points were held while Diane's eyes were in these pain-activating positions. As she did so, the pain in each area subsided and finally disappeared. On re-testing, Diane's muscles were now totally in balance.

A week later Diane was completely clear of all pain in her arms, legs and shoulders, and had only a slight twinge in the neck. She was instructed to put her neck in the position of pain and place her own hands on the ESR points, rotating her eyes until she felt her eyes flicker. At that point she should hold the position, and see whether the pain left her. This was entirely successful, and Diane was able to relieve her own pain.

From information supplied by Kay McCarroll, MC,
MIPC, DHP

HYPERTON-X
(HYPERTONIC MUSCLE RELEASE)

Hyperton-X is a gentle way of working with muscles which can benefit people with learning disorders, poor athletic performance, chronic pain, emotional problems, or colour and food sensitivities. It has been known to help people suffering from strokes, cerebral palsy, accident trauma, and general body pains, and can help bring about an overall improvement in general academic skills, co-ordination and confidence.

In 1982 Frank Mahony, a Californian TFH instructor, began working with junior-high school students (ages 12–14), using TFH concepts and other holistic principles to help poor readers. Noting the marked improvements in reading scores, he joined forces with Paul Dennison, founder of Educational Kinesiology, assisting him in Edu-K workshops in the USA and Berlin. He went on to bring out his own programme, Hyperton-X, as a separate and unique methodology. Several of Mahony's concepts regarding cerebro-spinal fluid self-correction and

In testing and correcting gifted athletes, Mahony established a definite correlation between the level of athletic performance and mental ability, hemispheric brain and energy systems integration, and the hypertonic state of muscles. He also acquired an understanding of the Sacro-Occipital-Technique (SOT), a chiropractic method, and its effect on cerebro-spinal fluid. Incorporating his TFH knowledge, he began to develop a method of detecting and correcting hypertonic muscles which had an effect on the sacrum and the occiput. By releasing these key muscles he was able to affect the flow of cerebro-spinal fluid, enhance the performance of the endocrine (glandular) system, release any neuro-muscular jamming (which blocks body/mind communication) and create a more harmonious holistic health system.

This technique uses muscle testing as a form of biofeedback, specifically to identify the hypertonic state of key muscles. Hyperton-X uses an indicator muscle, IM, to test the degree of stress when a specific muscle is in extension. Correction involves the client slowly activating the muscle towards contraction, while simultaneously breathing out. Releasing these hypertonic muscles enhances body/mind integration.

AN ATHLETE WITH CHRONIC PAIN

Bob, aged 38, was a fence-builder by profession, and also a keen athlete and football player. His activities had become limited by a pain in his mid and lower back and right hip, with shooting pains down both legs.

He had already had some chiropractic treatment, and medical X-rays showed that there was no misalignment in the vertebrae; however, there was a twist in the lumbar region, and one of his hips was higher than the other. Hyperton-X assessment

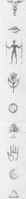

confirmed the X-ray findings, and found that the lumbar twist and imbalance were due to hypertonic muscles.

He was given a Touch For Health balance, and the hypertonic muscles were treated with gentle Hyperton-X breathing and stretching techniques, in order of priority. This released the tension. The muscles were then reprogrammed to improve communication between them and the brain. Follow-up treatments involved further Hyperton-X release.

Bob was completely free of pain within six months, and was able to carry on with his football training and heavy fencing work. He now has a regular bi-annual maintenance treatment to keep himself fit and active for work and for sport. In between these sessions he uses self-maintenance Hyperton-X exercises at home.

From information supplied by Kay McCarroll, MC,
MIPC, DHP

HEALTH KINESIOLOGY (HK)

Health Kinesiology was developed by Dr Jimmy Scott. It is concerned with finding and correcting physical, psychological and environmental stresses, taking into account not only the causes of a particular set of symptoms but also the processes which help to keep the problem going.

HK aims at removing old, inappropriate psychological patterns, correcting allergies and nutritional deficiencies, and working out individual programmes for diet, exercise, rest and play. It helps people to function more effectively in life, and also to make the necessary changes to improve their lifestyle.

Muscle testing is used to assess what is needed, and corrections include acupressure holding points and sometimes magnets, crystals, homoeopathic substances and essential oils. Sometimes the person is asked to think about something in particular, or touch a part of his or her body while the acupuncture points are held.

HK is also concerned with correcting problems of geopathic stress (harmful earth radiations) and electromagnetic pollution from computers, television sets, etc., and with removing drug and heavy metal residues from the system.

As the following case histories indicate, HK can be successful with a wide variety of conditions, and has treated successfully such diverse problems as agoraphobia, hay-fever, asthma, eczema, osteoarthritis and rheumatoid arthritis, dizziness, back problems, frozen shoulders, pre-menstrual tension, nail-biting, panic attacks, lack of self-confidence, Chronic Fatigue Syndrome, Candida Albicans, bronchitis and stress-related problems.

AN ALLERGY TO FISH

Sam, aged 67, had always had problems eating fish. His lips and throat would swell and he would ache as the food moved down his alimentary canal. In general he could avoid eating it, but after a meal out in which the cook had used a fish stock, Sam ended up in his usual sorry state, and resolved to do something about it.

The practitioner first worked to strengthen his immune system, and to correct a problem Sam had in metabolizing the mineral manganese. Careful muscle testing showed that he would be able to eat fish, starting initially with very small quantities, five and a half months later.

Six months after this one treatment Sam phoned, to say delightedly that he had eaten some fish several days before with no ill-effects at all. He was amazed that this long-standing problem had been resolved with a single, one-hour visit to a Health Kinesiologist.

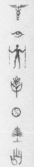

VERTIGO

Richard, 61, had suffered from vertigo for ten or fifteen years. His GP had diagnosed inner-ear damage caused by a flu virus, and had told him he would have to live with it.

Since Richard's job involved climbing trees, this was a real problem. Sometimes he had to lash himself to a tree to prevent himself falling off – fortunately he usually had some warning that the vertigo was about to start.

Most HK consultations last an hour, but Richard needed several short appointments rather than one long one. During these he was treated with magnets to help to re-balance his electromagnetic energy. He was also asked to visualize himself in vertigo-inducing situations while reflex points were held.

Two years later, Richard is basically symptom-free, and delighted with the results. Sometimes when he is very tired he experiences the warning sensation; when this happens he knows he has to ease up.

PSORIASIS

Rosemary had had psoriasis for five months, and was understandably anxious to prevent it from getting worse. Her small son's asthma had been treated successfully with HK, so she decided to try it, too.

Assessment found that Rosemary's liver and kidneys were not functioning as well as they should. This did not mean that she was likely to develop a serious illness, but without some help for these vital organs her psoriasis was unlikely to disappear.

In Rosemary's case, her low liver and kidney function were found to be related to stressful emotions. Her treatment involved her thinking about feelings that distressed her, such as sadness, anxiety, and fear of being useless, while the practitioner held the reflex points that would take the emotional charge out of these thoughts.

By the time she came for her second appointment, her skin was already almost clear. She decided to continue having HK for the arthritis she also suffered from, and her husband - who had had psoriasis for 40 years – also decided to try it. He, too, is now getting better through the use of similar techniques, together with magnet therapy.

From information supplied by Jane Thurnell-Read
MSc, Grad. IPM

CLINICAL KINESIOLOGY (CK)

Clinical Kinesiology is a highly complex and sophisticated system which is used mainly by health professionals trained in manipulative skills. It emphasizes the importance of good communication between various systems and parts of the body in the creation of good health. The ultimate case of noncommunication is cancer, where a sick area of the body is walled off from healthy tissues, preventing resolution of the problem.

Also known as Human BioDynamics (HBD), CK was the brainchild of the late Dr Alan Beardall, a chiropractor of great vision and intuition, from Utah, USA. He developed a number of revolutionary ideas that extended AK into new frontiers, many of which have been integrated into other systems of Kinesiology. An important example is the leg lock, also called the pause lock, which is a way of retaining in the whole body information acquired through muscle testing, in order to build on it. He also pioneered the technique of cumulative Two-pointing, in which chains of related facts can be discovered in their order of priority.

CK exploits the parallels between muscle testing in the human body and the electronic computer. Both are biphasic: a muscle is either strong or weak, while a computer circuit is either open or closed, on or off. In both cases, information is

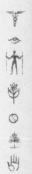

transmitted. Dr Beardall developed sophisticated ways of using the human 'bio-computer' both diagnostically and therapeutically. He also postulated that information is stored at different levels, some of it as if in files, and that the safest and most effective way of approaching a patient's problems is to deal with the superficial ('non-filed') problems before going to deeper-level ('filed') information.

Dr Beardall believed that pain (or any other symptom, physical or otherwise) is the body's way of communicating a need for change. If that requirement is satisfied, the person can progress along life's path in a positive and healthy direction. If the inner cry for help is ignored, the body will try to adapt, but at the price of decreased efficiency of function and less resistance to further stresses, which create an ever-steeper spiral into ill-health.

CK is a powerful tool for halting and reversing this spiral. It presents an efficient way for the body to choose the appropriate therapy at that time: chemical, structural, or emotional/ electromagnetic, and has enabled many practitioners successfully to treat patients with serious problems which they were previously unable to approach.

Dr Beardall was tragically killed in a road accident in November 1987. By then he had completed the bulk of a project listing every division of every muscle in the body, along with testing procedures and all the factors associated with each muscle, such as nerve supply, acupuncture meridians, associated organs, vertebral levels, cranial and foot bones, as well as neuro-lymphatic and neuro-vascular reflexes and specific nutritional requirements. Since his death a dozen further variations have arisen, as individual practitioners have applied their own expertise to the vista of possibilities he opened up.

There are two ways of selecting which area of therapy is required. One involves diagnostic points on the skull; the other uses arm positions or modes combined with an IM test. Dr Beardall also discovered and developed hand modes (see page 55) to determine appropriate treatment; in CK more than 1000 hand modes have been catalogued, some simple, some complex.

The structural therapy modes include established manipulative techniques, muscle work and cranio-sacral therapy, as well as many innovations developed by Dr Beardall and other experts. Electromagnetic treatment includes vibrational/energy medicines such as gems, flower and homoeopathic remedies and essential oils, and the manual treatment of acupuncture points.

Rigorous testing is carried out after treatment to ensure that the treatment or remedy has had the desired effect at all appropriate levels in all parts of the body. This involves testing arm and leg length, which must end up even. (It is surprising how often there is an imbalance between limb lengths at the first assessment.) Muscle groups in the neck and all four limbs are also tested.

In CK attention to body chemistry is important to the success of treating difficult or chronic problems. To meet this requirement, Dr Beardall developed his own range of synergistically-balanced nutritional supplements, which include all the trace elements and precursors needed to utilize them optimally.

The following case histories show how a variety of therapies are used in this complex but undoubtedly holistic form of therapy.

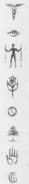

Wendy, 32, had two children, and had suffered from colitis for three-and-a-half years; it had appeared during her first pregnancy. During her second pregnancy it had recurred with a vengeance, and she had been treated with large doses of steroids. When she first saw an osteopath/Clinical Kinesiologist, she was still taking these, at a lower dose, together with another medical drug.

CK testing showed that she needed a nutritional support programme to help her combat multiple allergies. She was given a multi-vitamin and mineral supplement, RNA, and support for the adrenal glands. Flower Remedies were prescribed to help with an underlying emotional trauma, and various structural therapies were used to aid the blood flow to and out of the diseased tissues. Wendy improved steadily, and in less than five months had come off all her drugs.

Her right leg was shorter than the left, and she was given a heel lift to compensate. In the second phase of her treatment programme, detoxification of the bowel and liver enabled her body to 'hold' structural corrections aimed at equalizing her leg lengths.

She had a relapse when she became pregnant for a third time, but recovered with continued nutritional support and dietary management, along with cranio-sacral therapy. Four years after this she is still fit and healthy, and her leg lengths remain even.

SUB-FERTILITY

Kathy, 33, was a doctor's receptionist who had been trying to conceive for two-and-a-half years. She and her husband had had a range of tests, but nothing abnormal had been diagnosed. For six months she had been taking a drug to stimulate ovulation.

Although she was very fit and strong, CK testing showed several areas of endocrine imbalance. Differences in her leg lengths suggested a spleen meridian imbalance, associated with sugar metabolism problems which were affecting her immune system.

She was given caprylic acid salts (a natural antifungal) and probiotics to combat an overgrowth of candida in the gut which was affecting her uterus. Using hand modes, her liver was found to be interfering with her spleen and thymus, affecting both her immune and endocrine systems through the pituitary gland. This was dealt with through supplements which provided nutritional support to her liver.

The next step was to treat the way the muscles in Kathy's body had adapted to the above problems, which had caused weakness in her lateral hip muscles (which are associated with the ovaries). After structural work on these muscles, Vitamin E was recommended to support the function of her ovaries.

Six weeks later, six months after starting treatment, Kathy conceived. She needed a little pre-natal care, mainly in the form of keeping the craniosacral mechanism in balance. After the birth, both mother and baby were given cranial treatment. (Cranial treatment after birth can be very beneficial for any mother and baby.) Kathy then needed a little nutritional support in the form of a multi-mineral supplement designed to feed the autonomic nervous system.

At the time of writing the baby is nine months old, beautiful and healthy. His parents are delighted.

From information supplied by Ashley Robinson,
DO, MRO

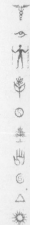

ADVANCED KINESIOLOGY

For well over a decade Dr Sheldon Deal has been presenting annual seminars world wide on Advanced Kinesiology. The material is a synthesis of research papers presented at the

annual ICAK conferences and Sheldon Deal's own research. He
selects and modifies the material for professional kinesiologists
and students most of whom do not belong to the ICAK and do
not have manipulative skills. This material now represents a
considerable body of knowledge and forms the basis for
advanced kinesiology training courses. It offers an alternative
to the Professional Kinesiology Practitioner (PKP) training
mentioned earlier in the chapter. One of the training organizations offering Advanced Kinesiology is the Academy of
Systematic Kinesiology (TASK), a British organization formed
by Brian Butler to educate the public in basic and Advanced
Kinesiology.

Brian Butler was a pioneer in bringing Touch For Health to
Europe in 1976. Systematic Kinesiology is the name he gave to
a training programme which teaches Balanced Health, based
on Touch For Health, and the intermediate and advanced
Kinesiology techniques taught by Dr Sheldon Deal.

The Academy syllabus teaches only Kinesiological procedures which are accepted as AK practice by the International
College of Applied Kinesiology (ICAK). These have been
described in Chapters 4, 5 and 6.

The following story is a good example of the holistic effects
of Advanced Kinesiology, and shows how balancing the whole
person can lead to important life changes.

THE TENSE LIBRARIAN

Paul, a librarian in his thirties, visited me complaining of neck
and shoulder pain, accompanied by numbness and tingling
down one side of his body. His GP had referred him to a neurol-
ogist, who had found nothing to account for his symptoms.

The Kinesiology assessment showed an imbalance in his neck
and shoulder muscles, as well as an imbalance between his
right- and left-brain hemispheres. During the assessment session

Paul mentioned that he was frustrated in his work; what he really wanted was to pursue an interest in alternative health, and to spend more time with his music. However, with a wife and a mortgage to maintain, he could see no way out of the work-trap.

Paul was literally finding his work a pain in the neck, and his frustration was causing him to hold certain muscles in constant tension. The fact that all his symptoms were affecting one side only was due to the imbalance between the brain hemispheres, resulting from over-use of his logical brain in his work and under-use of his creative hemisphere.

To resolve this, Paul needed to find a way of making changes in his working life which would allow him to develop his creative interests; it was also important for him to do this with the support of his wife, and to continue to earn enough to meet his financial commitments.

On the physical side, I corrected Paul's muscle imbalances, as well as advising him on ways of improving his diet and lifestyle. Through counselling, I helped him to identify a clear goal for himself; they then went on to develop short-term, medium-term and long-term plans that would give Paul more time and space for his creative side. As he began to appreciate that this was a real possibility, Paul developed a stronger belief in what he wanted to do, and who he wanted to be. He succeeded in negotiating a shorter working week with his employers, and as he embarked on his new life-plan his physical symptoms disappeared.

Two years later he is working very happily in a new job. He has completed his study in alternative therapy and is practising his music in his spare time. He has had no further health problems.

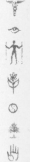

CONCLUSION

Unlike some systems of health care, which have a set body of knowledge, the muscle biofeedback tool provides almost unlimited scope for the development of Kinesiology. As well as the main branches, small branches have developed, and more are developing all the time. In time these may gain wider recognition.

Kinesiology is also a valuable tool for research into different aspects of health care, and may be utilized more widely in this area in the future.

SUMMARY CHART OF AK, TFH AND BRANCHES OF KINESIOLOGY

System/Branch	Practised by	What it is and does
AK: Applied Kinesiology	ICAK-trained chiropractors osteopaths, doctors, etc.	The parent of Kinesiology Developed from chiropractic, osteopathy, incorporates manipulative techniques. Deals with illness and disease as well as prevention.
TFH: Touch For Health/ FKP: Foundation Kinesiology Practitioner Balanced Health	Laypersons and health professionals	Synthesis of early basic AK material. A complete system which uses muscle testing and energy balancing for health enhancement/prevention. Based on John Thie's *Touch For Health*. Basic Kinesiology training.
PKP: Professional Kinesiology Practitioner	Health professionals, laypersons	Synthesis and adaptation of AK material prepared by Dr Bruce Dewe, offering advanced Kinesiology training. Has its own assessment procedures, e.g. finger modes, 'asking the body'.
Edu-K: Educational Kinesiology	Teachers, health professionals, laypersons	Specialized approach to mind/body integration, particularly as it affects learning, dyslexia, co-ordination, etc. Uses special exercises, movements, and many electrical and other energy corrections.

Three-in-One Concepts	Therapists, health professionals, laypersons	Focuses on emotional factors. Uses muscle biofeedback for age recession and Behavioural Barometer for identifying emotional states. Treats with Stress Defusion techniques (frontal-occipital holding)
BK: Biokinesiology	Health professionals, laypersons	Works on connections between emotions and organs and glands. Corrections include ESR plus eye rotations, positive affirmations, etc.
Hyperton-X	Sports therapists, health professionals, laypersons	Focuses on hypertonic (over-tight) muscles, releasing them through muscle activation and breathing. Promotes flow of cerebro-spinal fluid, improves body/mind integration and performance.
HK: Health Kinesiology	Health professionals, laypersons	Focuses on physical, psychological and environmental stresses. Assessment through muscle testing; corrections include holding acupressure and reflex points, using magnets, homoeopathic remedies, etc.
CK: Clinical Kinesiology	Osteopaths, chiropractors, health professionals	A sophisticated and complex extension of AK. Views the human system as a 'bio-computer'; uses hundreds of hand modes to access information from the body.
Advanced Kinesiology	Health professionals, laypersons	Synthesis of AK material prepared by Dr Sheldon Deal for non-medical, non-manipulative health professionals. Annual updates by Dr Deal of latest AK research.

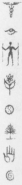

KINESIOLOGY AND OTHER FIELDS

K inesiology can be a truly valuable adjunct to other therapies and branches of health care, for a number of reasons. First, it provides a genuinely holistic approach, which many therapies do not; secondly, muscle testing as a biofeedback tool can be an invaluable aid in the selection of treatments and remedies; thirdly, it offers a practical way of working with the dimension of subtle energy and a means of using that in assessment and treatment.

This chapter gives examples of the success of Kinesiology in a variety of fields. Since Kinesiology is still in the throes of expansion it is not as yet used by vast numbers of therapists. However, we hope that readers will gain an idea of what Kinesiology can achieve, and that professionals in other fields will be inspired to add it to their skills.

Meanwhile, not all practitioners who claim to be using Kinesiology are in fact doing so. For muscle testing to be an accurate diagnostic tool a number of factors have to be checked, and untrained therapists inevitably get unreliable results, on occasions giving Kinesiology a bad name. So, if you visit someone who claims, for example, to be using Kinesiology to test for allergies, and only uses a single muscle test, his or her advice may be far from accurate. For Kinesiology to be applied

correctly in any therapeutic discipline, very precise procedures
must be followed.

The Foundation Kinesiology Practitioner training course provides a thorough foundation training for practitioners and students in other fields.

KINESIOLOGY AS AN ADJUNCT TO HOLISTIC MEDICINE

The response of many doctors to their first brush with Kinesiology is similar to that of Dr Rodney Adeniyi-Jones, who was at the time working in a research laboratory in a teaching hospital. When he first saw muscle testing his reaction was 'not only disbelief, but complete disregard.'

In the UK, Kinesiology is so unrelated to medical training that most British doctors are unaware of its existence. This is a great pity, for its incorporation into medical diagnosis and treatment could reduce National Health Service outlay on expensive drugs and prolonged tests. It could also save patients a good deal of anguish through misdiagnosis or the limitations of conventional medicine in dealing with stress, chronic pain and many other health problems – especially since few GPs and even fewer consultants look at all sides of the Triad of Health. However, British doctors are becoming increasingly interested in the notion of holistic medicine, and increasingly open-minded towards the use of complementary therapies such as acupuncture and homoeopathy.

In the case of Dr Adeniyi-Jones, he eventually attended a Touch For Health course, and discovered for himself how well muscle testing can work. Two years later, when he made contact with ICAK, heard George Goodheart lecture, and explored the literature, he realized that there was a body of detailed, well-referenced research behind the techniques of Applied Kinesiology. He writes:

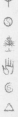

This was, to me, an immense relief, and it gave me the information I needed to decide whether I could really take Kinesiology *seriously*: I could. Applied Kinesiology is now a pivotal part of my practice.

Integration is the key to therapeutic success with difficult illnesses. Complex homoeopathy, clinical nutrition, phytotherapy (the use of herbs) and auriculotherapy (ear acupuncture) fit easily into the treatment system, along with cranial and pelvic adjustment, emotional support and neurological integration.

It has become clear to me that every form of treatment can affect all sides of the Triad of Health – but nothing apart from Kinesiology treats all sides in such a direct, effective, balanced manner.

Because the muscle test is not 'completely objective' [that is, the Kinesiologist is part of the test] I am happy to be able to use laboratory and other tests in conjunction with it, particularly in serious and dangerous illnesses. But in such situations, the results obtained when treatment is integrated by Kinesiology are spectacular.[1]

One of Dr Adeniyi-Jones's patients was a woman suffering from a whole range of painful problems.

INTEGRATED TREATMENT

Jane was a company director of 35 who had had severe asthma since the age of 17, which had not benefited from a change of diet following allergy tests. At 30 she had developed endometriosis; medication for this brought on depression, acne and a weight problem. At 34 she developed arthritis; medication for this aggravated her asthma.

[1] A copy of Dr Adeniyi-Jones' article, 'The Muscle Test – How Does it Work?' can be obtained by contacting Dr Adeniyi-Jones (see 'Medicine' in Appendix B).

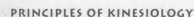

It was at this point that she sought holistic treatment from Dr Adeniyi-Jones. Within four months of starting integrated treatment with Applied Kinesiology, her joint pains, back pain, foot swelling and low energy had disappeared. Her energy level returned to normal, her periods became lighter and less painful, and her asthma steadily improved.

Nurses are beginning to take an interest in Kinesiology and Touch For Health in Britain, while in the USA there are nurses who have trained in TFH and incorporate it into hospital treatment to relieve stress and pain. They also show patients how they can use self-help techniques, even in hospital beds.

Hypnotherapist Christine Baldwin originally used Kinesiology while working in hospital as an Occupational Therapist. After completing only the basic level of Touch For Health she was able to use it to relieve muscle pain in stroke patients, and to increase the power in weakened muscles. Occupational Therapists, she says, 'consider themselves pretty holistic in their approach to patients. We always take into consideration a person's mental and physical state as well as their home environment, job, family relationships and so on. A Kinesiologist does all this, plus assessing chemical/nutritional factors and environmental factors such as electro-pollution and geopathic stress.'

A few British dentists are beginning to practise 'holistic dentistry', seeing their patients as more than a set of teeth, and incorporating Kinesiology into their work. One of them writes:

The use of Kinesiology is as relevant to dentistry as any other branch of health care. Apart from it being a system of diagnosis, it is a system of checking the correctness of the treatment prescribed. In other words, the success of the treatment prescribed can be ascertained in advance rather than on a trial-and-error basis.

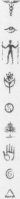

The treatment to which I am referring is an expanded form of dentistry which one could call holistic dentistry. It is equally appropriate in basic dentistry, but when used to assess and improve the whole sense of well-being of patients it assumes a more important role. Kinesiology can also be used for assessing and checking the need for nutritional supplementation. By nutrition, I do not mean drugs; I mean substances that we need to support and maintain life.

KINESIOLOGY AND MANIPULATIVE THERAPIES

As we have seen, Kinesiology originated within chiropractic, and is becoming more widely used not only by American but also by British chiropractors, as well as by some osteopaths and physiotherapists. Its use in manipulative therapies widens the choices available to practitioners; as a physiotherapist says, 'It presents a superb means of being able to evaluate and balance the body systems in a truly holistic, non-invasive and non-confrontational way … and to evaluate the effects of the therapy.'

CHIROPRACTIC

Chiropractic is a manipulative system offering a wide choice of techniques. Muscle testing, says Richard Cook, a chiropractor member of ICAK, takes the guesswork out of practice:

No longer are we 'pop and pray' merchants. We have at our disposal a sophisticated machine – the human body – which shows the answers if we ask the right questions. We can determine what to adjust, when to adjust, how to adjust, and whether the correction has worked. The body will show up problems in a preferential order – that is, in the way it would prefer to be fixed.

If that is respected, although it may be time-consuming, the improvements are well worth the wait.

Chiropractors correct mainly structural faults, but to be a complete practitioner in today's health care forum one has to be able to understand nutritional and chemical problems, as well as emotional traumas. With AK we have the means to work in all these areas, and often, using natural and relatively simple methods bring the patient back to a state of robust health.

CHRONIC BACK PAIN

A young man of 23 had been suffering low back pain for two years, with recurrent severe twinges mainly in the left leg, accompanied by some numbness. He did not know what had brought it on, except for a possible sprain after windsurfing. Physiotherapy had helped to some extent, but he was still experiencing constant dull pain in the buttock and thigh.

Chiropractic findings revealed a postural shift to the left, a degree of dural torque [a twist in the dura, the sheath protecting the spinal cord], and a short left leg. Standard diagnostic techniques, including X-rays, provided little information as to the cause of the trouble. Using AK the low back muscles were checked for integrity, and Therapy Localization showed that the left sacro-iliac joint needed adjustment. This was done, using specific chiropractic techniques which brought about a dramatic strengthening of the weak left hamstring. Further manipulation improved the general mobility of the patient, and the dull ache was dramatically reduced.

After four treatment sessions the young man made a full recovery.

Very often the cause of bodily pain is not found at the site of the pain. In the following case history, a jaw problem was contributing to pains in the patient's arm and shoulder.

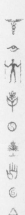

A professional singer of 46 had had pain in her left shoulder and arm for ten years, and it had begun to disturb her sleep. She had been deaf in her right ear since having mumps at the age of one; recently she had noticed slight tinnitus in her good ear.

X-rays of the cervical (neck) area of her spine showed that two vertebrae were misaligned, causing pressure on a disc. AK testing showed where there was muscle weakness, and where her neck needed adjusting. In addition, the practitioner noted that the woman had a jaw problem with a cross-bite and abnormal wear on her teeth on the front left side. She admitted to bruxism (tooth-grinding), which could relate to the noises in her ear.

Using Therapy Localization to the jaw joints, it was found that she had a major jaw problem, and that chewing caused stress to the rest of her body. The practitioner corrected these problems using special spindle cell muscle techniques (muscle reprogramming). After this treatment her sleeping improved, the tension in her jaw was relieved, and her arm pain disappeared completely.

McTimoney Chiropractor Isobel Stevenson practises and teaches Kinesiology, and has trained in cranio-sacral therapy. She finds that muscle testing is not only useful to her, but also to her clients. She comments, 'After adjusting the spine, or the pelvis, and so on, there is suddenly a big change in muscle strength. This gives the person very direct feedback that the treatment has been effective.'

The following is a good example of the holistic possibilities of combining chiropractic and Kinesiology. In conventional medicine the patient might have been referred to a rheumatologist, orthopaedic surgeon or physiotherapist for one set of symptoms, and to a gastro-intestinal specialist for another. In the event, the combination of chiropractic and Kinesiology covered all her problems.

A retired nurse of 60 had a bruised feeling in her ribs, a stiff, crackly neck, an aching left hip and a left ankle that ached and tended to swell. She had had her gall-bladder removed some 15 years before. Now she had been suffering from indigestion for several months, very loose stools for three years, and haemorrhoids. She also had an occasional sharp pain in the right lower abdomen. Her doctor had treated her indigestion with antacids.

Kinesiology assessment revealed an ileocecal valve (ICV) problem, and imbalances in her stomach, small intestine and large intestine. Prioritizing showed that the ICV problem was primarily structural; she had some misalignments in her lumbar spine, and the nerves in that area connect with the ileocecal valve.

She first had two sessions of McTimoney chiropractic. After these, her neck was much better, the aching and swelling in her ankle had gone and the pain in her ribs was absent for most of the time. Her bowel movements were still soft, but only happened once a day instead of four or five times; the piles were improving.

At the third session, Kinesiology testing revealed a hiatus hernia at a subclinical level; that is, at too early a stage to be picked up by medical diagnosis. The primary imbalance involved showed up as chemical. Food sensitivity testing showed that the woman was primarily sensitive to dairy products, which she agreed to cut out for a time.

She continued having chiropractic treatments, and was much more careful with her diet. A weakness in her abdominal muscles was also found, and she was shown how to treat them at home with gentle exercise and by massaging specific Kinesiology points.

After four months there had been a dramatic improvement all round, and the woman's digestion and bowels were functioning normally, unless she ate something that upset her.

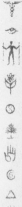

It was not necessary to treat either the ICV or the hiatus hernia directly. The structural work and the dietary changes simply removed them from the picture by clearing them indirectly.

OSTEOPATHY

Osteopathy, like chiropractic, is primarily aimed at correcting structural problems, and uses manipulation and soft-tissue work. Both believe that treatment of the spine can improve overall health as well as treating musculo-skeletal problems.

Christopher Smith is a Registered Osteopath, a member and Diplomate of ICAK and a leading authority and teacher of AK in Britain and Europe. He also uses cranial therapy. As the following cases show, his work covers a much broader field than simply dealing with the spine, joints and muscles.

BACKACHE AND SUB-FERTILITY

Mrs M., a secretary aged 30, was suffering from constant lower backache radiating to both sides. She had so far been unable to conceive. She had also been in two road accidents, resulting in whiplash injuries.

AK assessment found that she had a pelvic torque (twist), a weak piriformis muscle (an important muscle in the hip), and needed cranial treatment. She also needed Vitamin E.

After several osteopathic treatments, including cranio-sacral therapy, Mrs M. was free of back pain and has remained so. And, although the treatment was not directly aimed at treating sub-fertility, five months later she became pregnant.

When a child is hyperactive, it is often assumed that diet is to blame, and some unfortunate children have been put on near-starvation regimes by people suspecting allergens in just about every food. Kinesiology, however, is invaluable in pin-pointing not the most obvious, but the most effective treatment.

This child was suffering from headaches, insomnia and hyperactivity. His mother related that his birth had been difficult; the labour was protracted, and forceps had been used.

AK assessment found a compression of a bone in the child's skull; after treating this his sleep pattern improved immediately, and follow-up treatments substantially reduced his hyperactivity. His sleep became normal, and he had no more headaches.

EXAM NERVES

A girl of 16 was suffering acute anxiety about her forthcoming GCSE exams. An AK assessment led to treatment with the Bach Flower Remedy Oak, Emotional Stress Release, stimulation of an acupuncture point, and Vitamin B supplementation.

After one treatment the girl was more relaxed at the prospect of her exams. One further treatment was given on the day before the exams started. She sat them free of panic, with her memory working perfectly, and she passed nine subjects.

PHYSIOTHERAPY

Sheila Cozens, a Chartered Physiotherapist, began looking into complementary therapies because she was aware that there were certain groups of patients who had remained uninfluenced by conventional therapies alone. They were generally people with chronic problems, who often presented with complex signs and symptoms. However, like other medically-trained practitioners, when she first saw a demonstration of Touch For Health she found it hard to accept that muscle testing could provide information about the state of a person's well-being. In the light of her physiotherapy education and experience, this concept created some conflict for her.

However, when she herself was balanced, she could detect differences in her system while she was being worked on, and

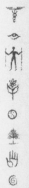

felt substantially different afterwards. The following day, she experienced a marked reduction in symptoms she had been experiencing consistently for some time, which had not responded to other treatment.

Sheila has now trained in Kinesiology, which she finds 'a very flexible system which can be used in many different circumstances for different kinds of problems.' She uses it to help chronic cases, as well as people with shorter-term problems, and finds more and more people coming back periodically for 'tune-up' sessions, while some like to be worked on from a purely preventive point of view.

AN IMMEDIATE CURE

An aerobics instructor of 36 developed a pain in her right hamstring area, with no known cause. She was due to run a marathon in two days' time, and was anxious to be well. Her GP had looked at her right leg and diagnosed a torn hamstring. Kinesiology assessment, however, showed that the problem had a different cause.

Muscle testing showed that the priority was the ICV. This was corrected using Kinesiology, and she was shown how to stimulate the correction points for herself. She was also given some dietary advice. She was asked to come back the next day to re-test the correction.

The woman had recovered and was running again before she came for her next session. She continued well enough to compete successfully in the race.

DENTISTRY

Dentistry is not usually classed as a 'manipulative therapy'; in fact it can have negative effects on the joints of the jaw and skull. Dental work, particularly if it is prolonged and painful, can also cause a good deal of stress. In addition it can affect the delicate balance of the jaw and neck, with reverberating effects on other parts of the body. However, some dentists are becoming aware of these effects, and are training in both Kinesiology and cranial/cranio-sacral therapy, which can also be of great benefit to their patients.

For example, the temperomandibular joint (TMJ), the jaw joint near the ear, plays a very important role in structural balance. Stress in this area caused by dental work often corrects itself, but it can be helpful to have it corrected by a Kinesiologist. Dentists who practise Kinesiology will do this automatically, but too few dental practitioners have a knowledge of these connections, as the following story shows.

LEG PAIN AFTER DENTISTRY

Gill, aged 43, suddenly developed an ache in her right calf muscle which she could not account for. It bothered her when she sat or lay down, and was bad enough to affect her sleep. An osteopath was unable to find the cause, and suspected a blood clot. Gill's GP, too, was unable to diagnose the cause. At the same time Gill was feeling 'fluey', tired, depressed and lethargic, and was suffering digestive problems, with flatulence and loss of appetite.

After a week the pain also affected her back, and she had a migraine one night, something she had not had since childhood. About three weeks after the pain started she attended a Touch For Health workshop. The person working with her found and worked on an ICV problem, and she was recommended to go to a chiropractor-Kinesiologist. She saw him next day, and he found it difficult at first to pin down what was wrong. He confirmed that there was an ICV problem, but that this would not stay 'fixed'; there seemed to be another priority.

Finally he pin-pointed a TMJ problem, and asked her if she had had any dental treatment lately. A month before she had in fact

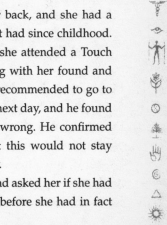

had two prolonged dental sessions, involving getting two crowns fitted and a root-filling, during which she had spent an hour at a time with her mouth wide open.

After the TMJ had been corrected the muscle ache subsided, as did all Gill's other symptoms.

Richard Sudworth, an holistic dentist who uses Kinesiology, writes:

> The relationship of the jaw joint to the rest of the skeleton cannot be emphasized enough. What goes on in the jaw joint is profoundly related to the structure and function of the neck and lower back. Correction of the wrongly positioned jaw joint can be assessed and checked with Kinesiology. This is the only way of consistently and accurately deciding on the best physiological position, which will make that patient feel and function better. This is why Kinesiology is so valuable with patients who complain of headaches, lack of well-being, bizarre aches and pains and, most critically of all, those who feel they have been abandoned as malingerers.
>
> Kinesiology can also be used for assessing the suitability of various filling materials. Some people react unfavourably to the insertion of mercury amalgams. It would be unwise to replace this material until you know that the substitute will be physiologically acceptable to that patient. This can be done easily with Kinesiology.

Muscle testing can be used to check individual teeth when the cause of a toothache is not immediately clear; and also to check the bite after treatment. It can in fact be used at any point in the course of dental treatment to assess what further work needs to be done, and afterwards to evaluate whether the treatment really is complete. Anyone who can go to a dentist trained in Kinesiology is very fortunate.

Many occupations have particular hazards, from the repetitive strain injury prevalent among word-processor operators to the neck and back problems suffered by people who drive long distances. Elizabeth Andrews, author of *Muscle Management* for keen sports people (Thorsons, 1991) is a Kinesiologist and chiropractor. She is also an experienced professional string-player, and her particular understanding of musicians' problems has brought many orchestral players to her clinic.

Simply playing an instrument can, over the years, cause distortions in the body, particularly instruments that are played to one side, such as violins, or brass and wind instruments which put pressure on the mouth and therefore the jaw area. In addition there are many tensions in the life of musicians which are not evident to concert audiences; working in cramped, uncomfortable conditions, living on junk food out of suitcases when on tour, having to play music they dislike – or music they do like, for the fiftieth time.

Most problems are cleared in four sessions, starting with a general chiropractic treatment to relieve pain and re-balance the body as far as possible, followed by a Kinesiology assessment to the main postural muscles and the problem areas. At the second session specific problems are looked at in greater depth; during the third session issues of stress and nutrition are assessed. (Nutrition can be very important to players; sugar, for instance, can weaken the spleen meridian, which connects with the muscles in the hand and forearm.) The fourth session ensures that the person is now fit to carry on.

The treatment often includes examining how the person holds his or her instrument, and suggesting ways of doing so with less strain and distortion, together with specific self-help techniques which can be practised during rehearsals. One violinist was helped with her low back pain by putting furniture

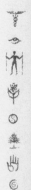

blocks under the back legs of her seat, tilting it forward to produce better posture – something that any desk-worker could
find useful. She was also shown how to massage the points that
would strengthen her abdominal muscles – something she
could do in free moments during rehearsals.

A VIOLINIST WITH CARPAL TUNNEL SYNDROME

Carpal tunnel syndrome is an injury caused by over-use; the
tendon in the wrist becomes inflamed causing great pain. It is
quite common in women in the late months of pregnancy.
Medical treatment usually consists of strapping it up and resting
it, or surgery. In the case of a violinist, this condition gives rise to
real anxiety for one's livelihood.

Sarah had overworked her wrist playing in a Wagner season,
and could no longer play without a lot of pain, and sensations
of pins and needles. Assessment found that the muscles in her
forearm and hand were reactive to each other: that is, the balance
between them was upset and the muscles were working
against one another instead of in co-operation. (See Muscle
Reprogramming, page 72.)

In this case, however, the trouble originated in the nerves in
Sarah's neck area, and the muscles of her neck and shoulders
were worked on. She was advised to stop playing for a short time
to allow the inflammation to subside. She was shown a point on
her ribs that she could stimulate to strengthen the area, and was
recommended nutritional support.

At the end of four sessions, Sarah was able to start gently
playing again. Since there is always a risk that an injury like this
can recur, she was recommended to come back regularly for
preventive treatment.

Jack had been in pain for some time, and had been advised to have an operation. Kinesiology muscle testing found that the root cause of the problem was his embouchure, that is, the way he arranged his mouth round the reed when playing.

The connection between the jaw and sciatica is explained by the fact, taught in Advanced Kinesiology, that some bones in the body will 'imitate' others. The sacrum, the shield-like bone at the base of the spine, is similar in shape to the bone at the back of the skull, and they tend to mimic one another.

In Jack's case, tightening his lips to play caused a jamming in his jaw joint, which in turn caused a jamming in his cranial bones, which was reflected in the bones at the base of his spine, creating pressure on his sciatic nerve. An operation to the lower back was unlikely to have solved his problem. Using Kinesiology to find out where the trouble started was the beginning of Jack's cure.

Liz Andrews is also a keen golfer, and so knows from both stage and green what it means to perform 'under fire'. As well as musicians, dancers and other entertainers often pop in for a check-up before important auditions. A typical example was June, a 25 year-old dancer.

A DANCER WITH AN ANKLE INJURY

June was seriously thinking of giving up her stage career because an old, recurring injury would not clear up despite a specialist's attention, and exercise. She had landed awkwardly after a leap, fracturing her foot. It had healed well and nothing showed up on X-ray, yet it had let her down again and again, usually when it mattered most. Now she had lost confidence.

Her foot and leg muscles were balanced, and the shock absorbers re-set. She was rebalanced while hopping on one leg, and finally she was placed in the position of the original injury.

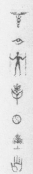

Further muscle imbalance showed up which was de-traumatized and balanced with ESR (see page 88).

She returned to dance class delighted, and despite warnings to go carefully, enthusiastically danced flat out. A week later she rang in distress to say the ankle was still not quite right. This time, on examination the priority was a hip misalignment, originally caused by over-doing the splits as a child. When this was corrected she had no further trouble.

This is a good example of the value of prioritizing, following what the body wants in the order it wants it – in June's case the foot disorder was priority, and the hip misalignment secondary. Most chiropractors would have treated the hip first, but in this case her body had adapted to that, and appropriately for a dancer – wanted the foot fixed first.

KINESIOLOGY AS AN AID TO NUTRITIONAL AND HERBAL REMEDIES

Kinesiology can be very useful to health practitioners who need to prescribe specific remedies, diets or nutritional supplements. The ability to balance a persons's energies adds a further dimension to any treatment, while recommending self-help techniques empowers people to be actively involved in their own healing process.

NUTRITIONAL THERAPY

We receive so much contradictory advice about nutrition today that it's easy to end up quite confused. The fact is that although there are broad nutritional guidelines which are true for most people, we are all individuals, with individual needs. Kinesiology is very helpful in finding out not only what an individual needs, but also how his or her needs can vary at different times.

In 1984 Diana Church, a qualified pharmacist of 13 years' standing, learned through personal experience how much one's health can be improved by changing one's diet and taking the right natural supplements. She studied nutrition, and in 1986 became a nutritional therapist, recommending vitamins and minerals as an aid to healing rather than as simple dietary supplements. However, she knew no way of finding out exactly which form of vitamins was needed for each particular client, or in what combinations, and had to work out each client's programme largely by trial and error.

In 1987 she discovered Kinesiology, and incorporated it into her practice with great success. It not only enables her to detect which vitamins and minerals each person needs, but also in what combinations. This has proved to be a great advantage and, she comments, very cost-effective for her clients, as well as improving their health rapidly. Moreover, she can now treat the whole body in a more balanced way.

Age is no barrier to recovering health through Kinesiology and good nutrition, as the following story shows.

A NATURAL ANSWER TO BOWEL PROBLEMS

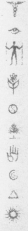

A garage forecourt attendant of 61 had a number of uncomfortable symptoms. He had frequent, loose bowel motions, and was unable to eat a range of 'healthy' foods, including most vegetables and wholemeal bread. He was suffering from lower back pain, stiff knees and elbows, and felt constantly tired, tense and snappy. His doctor had previously diagnosed colitis, for which he had prescribed a drug.

Kinesiology assessment found a severe vitamin and mineral imbalance, together with an ICV problem. Another valve in his bowels was also malfunctioning. These were corrected through

Kinesiology, and a nutritional programme was drawn up to restore the vitamin and mineral imbalance.

Two weeks later, at his second session, the client felt better than he had for years. He had had no pain since the first consultation. After that he returned monthly for regular Kinesiology balancing, and has maintained his good health. He has plenty of energy, can eat most vegetables, his bowels are working as they should, and he is free of pain.

While holistic doctors and natural therapists often look these days for an emotional cause to physical problems, body chemistry can also influence the emotions.

DIET AND STRESS

A woman clerk of 42 was unable to work; she was suffering from a fuzzy head, tiredness, pre-menstrual tension, and a total lack of confidence or motivation. She had formerly enjoyed running, but it was no longer a pleasure to her. Her doctor, diagnosing depression, had treated her with an anti-depressant drug, which had not helped her.

She was found to be suffering from a vitamin and mineral imbalance, including a severe zinc deficiency. Her adrenal glands (the stress-handling glands of the body) were exhausted, and her blood-sugar levels were swinging outside the normal range. A programme of supplements was recommended to help her adrenals and balance her vitamin and mineral levels, together with regular monthly Kinesiology treatment.

The improvement was rapid; the woman's depression lifted; she returned to work, and within six weeks was feeling so good that other people commented on the difference. She can now run long distances, and her pre-menstrual tension and depression have disappeared, even when she is under stress.

Aromatherapy is an ancient approach to healing which uses massage combined with precisely chosen essential oils whose smell and chemistry trigger a healing response in the body. Each essential oil has healing properties, and one of the skills of the aromatherapist is to find the right oils, or combination of oils, for each person. Muscle testing, in conjunction with other diagnostic information, can be used to help select the most appropriate essential oils, and Kinesiology correction techniques can be integrated into the aromatherapy massage to enhance the treatment.

The muscle-meridian/organ-gland assessment gives the therapist additional information, not only about the state of the person's energy and how that relates to his or her health, but also about subtle energy imbalances which could lead to health problems.

IRRITABLE BOWEL SYNDROME

Maureen, aged 30, was a divorced marketing consultant who visited aromatherapist Jacqueline Taylor suffering from irritable bowel syndrome (IBS), which included pain and constipation; she had had the condition for over five years. She was also suffering from nervous tension.

Combined Kinesiology/Aromatherapy assessment found a number of muscle imbalances, including ones related to the large intestine, together with a need to look at Maureen's diet, which included six cups of coffee and two or three glasses of alcohol a day. Maureen was also found to be suffering both from emotional stress related to her divorce some years earlier and post-operative trauma resulting from an operation for a prolapsed colon.

She was given four sessions of aromatherapy massage, including activation of specific Kinesiology reflexes. Muscle testing showed that she needed different oils at each session. She was

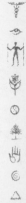

also encouraged to use essential oils in her bath at home, to change her diet, reduce her alcohol intake and increase her consumption of water. To help her deal with her emotional problems, Emotional Stress Release was used, together with visualization.

During the second session Maureen was able to relax very deeply, and by the third she had no more pain or discomfort in the bowel area, and felt stronger emotionally. By session four her bowel movements were normal, her stomach was no longer bloated, she was free of pain, and muscles that had originally tested weak were now strong. She had had one day of discomfort after an evening out which included alcohol; this confirmed to her that the change of diet was necessary. She enjoys her treatments very much, and goes back regularly to maintain her progress and reinforce her new sense of well-being.

MEDICAL HERBALISM

Medical herbalism is an increasingly popular form of natural therapy; in the right hands it offers a safe alternative to medical drugs, without the dangers of side-effects. Herbalism works by affecting the body's chemistry and, as we have seen, Kinesiology is highly useful in testing all aspects of body chemistry, and correcting related problems.

Qualified Medical Herbalists have a wide range of herbs to choose from, and there is often a choice of herbs to treat specific symptoms. Kinesiology can help the herbalist to select the most effective herb, or combination of herbs. At the same time, other aspects of the person can be addressed, such as balancing the emotions, or right-/left-brain co-ordination.

POST-OPERATIVE TRAUMA

A schoolgirl of 17 went to see Daphne Benjamin, a member of the Institute of Medical Herbalists; she had had constant sore throats since having her tonsils out four years earlier. Her GP had given her antibiotics. On assessment she was found to be suffering from nervous tension, and possibly from a viral infection. However, the appropriate herbal remedy did not have the desired effect, indicating that a virus was not the root cause of the problem.

Next, the emotional aspect of the girl's health was addressed, using Health Kinesiology techniques of brain, body and energy integration. Holding her ESR points enabled the patient to identify her fears. It emerged that she had been suffering from a fear of suffocation since the time when a mask had been put over her face for her tonsillectomy operation. The ESR treatment helped to clear this. She was given a tonic herbal mixture to boost her system generally.

A month later, the girl reported that she was clear of sore throats. Whether or not there had been a viral infection, clearing the emotional trauma enabled her body to free itself of sore throats. Some time later her throat problem had still not recurred.

COUNSELLING, PSYCHOTHERAPY AND LIFESTYLE

The emotional side of the Triad of Health is receiving much more attention these days, in the fields of both complementary and orthodox medicine. There is a greater understanding of the influence of the mind on health – particularly but not exclusively in the realms of energy/vibrational medicine – and less inclination for practitioners to tell people to 'pull themselves together and get on with it'.

Emotional stress can cause physical pain and tension, which can be relieved by muscle balancing. Chemical factors can contribute to emotional stress: coffee and sugar are often major parts of the diet of people who are depressed or tense, as most people don't realize that coffee is actually a stimulant which can increase stress, while an excessive intake of sugar can

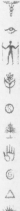

contribute to mood swings. Thus a change in diet can in itself reduce stress levels.

Using Kinesiology, the therapist can tell through the body's biofeedback just what effect an emotional issue is having – even one that the client may be not fully aware of – and techniques such as Emotional Stress Release, and emotional balancing together with energy balancing, can help people to face and cope with their problems.

COUNSELLING

People usually seek counselling when there is a particular issue they would like to understand better, or to change. It may be a situation in life, such as difficulties in their marriage or work, or some pattern of behaviour or attitude, such as an addiction, or low self-esteem.

Counselling combined with Kinesiology provides an extremely effective way of dealing with these issues, and usually in a much shorter period than might be involved in having psychotherapy only. Kinesiology has integrated some techniques from Neuro-Linguistic Programming (NLP), which provides methods with which to expand people's options in the way they think about things, thus creating more choices in life. Techniques include setting positive goals or outcomes (described in Chapter 6), the use of specific eye movements as in Biokinesiology, age regression, techniques for changing perceptions of the past, and, of course, emotional stress release.

Many of the Kinesiology corrections described in earlier chapters can be helpful in dealing with the kinds of emotional imbalance that are often brought to counsellors. The comprehensive list below gives some idea of the scope available. Needless to say, a counsellor would select very carefully which would be appropriate to the client concerned.

- Creating well-formed goals or outcomes (i.e. identifying what you want, instead of focusing on what you don't want. See Chapter 6, page 82)
- Emotional Stress Release
- Right-/Left-brain hemisphere integration
- Age regression
- Emotional balancing using the Law of Five Elements
- Bach Flower Remedies
- Psychological reversal
- Phobia cure
- Resolving conflicts in beliefs, such as are often found in addiction.

Self-help techniques are also given to empower people to help themselves. These include Emotional Stress Release, attention to diet, Bach Flower Remedies, and exercises to promote right-/left-brain co-ordination, all of which help to create and maintain emotional balance.

I myself work as a Kinesiologist and NLP practitioner/counsellor, and some sessions with clients move more towards counselling than energy balancing, depending on the client's needs at the time.

DEPRESSION

Helen, a 39-year-old teacher, and single parent, came to see me. She had been suffering from fatigue and depression since the birth of her son 12 years earlier and had been an out-patient of a Psychiatric Department for 10 years. She also had a pain in her upper chest, and irregularities in her menstrual cycle.

My assessment was that she was in a negative loop. For the last 12 years she had been focusing on her problems; she had never considered a positive outcome for herself, and had no concept of what that might be. The pain in her upper chest was partly due

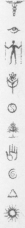

to muscle imbalances. By using an IM test with my hand in her energy field I found that it was also partly due to an emotional imbalance in that area of her subtle energy body. Her meridian energy was quite unbalanced, and her diet needed attention.

The first and most important part of the whole treatment was to help her find a direction, and discover what she wanted for herself, how she wanted to be, and to have a real sense of what that would be like. She achieved this in the first couple of sessions; her deep depression lifted and has never returned. The pain in her chest was cleared by balancing muscles in that area and giving healing in the energy field over the pain. Regular energy balancing harmonized her body's energies, and as a result her fatigue lessened considerably (she has a demanding job). Her menstrual cycle is now regular.

She has helped herself to maintain a more balanced perspective on life between sessions by balancing her brain hemispheres with Cross Crawl and eye movements, and by using Emotional Stress Release.

During the course of treatment I also used other techniques such as age regression and emotional balancing. The major changes were achieved in five or six sessions.

Helen is now happy and coping well with the demands of her busy life. She continues to come for sessions from time to time, knowing she can come when she needs extra support in time of need. She has had no need to return to the Psychiatric Department.

MANAGEMENT TRAINING

An increasing number of companies and organizations in the private and public sectors are recognizing the value of putting resources into the care and well-being of their staff. Professor Cary Cooper, a world expert in stress-management at work, has shown that it pays companies to look after their staff's psychological needs; happy employees mean fewer lost working hours and, of course, higher profits. Kinesiology can offer fast, effective ways to set goals, improve communication, performance and creativity, reduce stress and create harmony at both individual and group levels.

One of the most useful tools in Kinesiology is goal-setting. The guidelines come from NLP, and are simple to apply to individuals and groups. Muscle testing is also an amazingly effective demonstration tool for trainers. It can be used to show the physical and mental effects of poor communication, poor diet and disorganized electrical circuits (i.e. poor body/mind integration); self-help corrections can be taught for all of these.

In communication skills training, muscle testing can be used to show the instantaneous physical effects that spoken words can have on people. For instance, words like 'but' and 'should' will have a weakening effect on most people, whereas using the words 'and' and 'would like' in similar sentences strengthens most people. Although we know that praise feels good and criticism doesn't, few people realize just how profound an effect either can have on their whole physiology until it is vividly demonstrated.

Many Kinesiology techniques used in private practice can be usefully applied in work settings: assessing and correcting electromagnetic faults which cause disorganization in the body/mind, improving the communication between the eyes and the brain, and between the ears and the brain, and brain hemisphere integration for clear and balanced thinking.

Chemical factors that adversely affect performance can also be demonstrated, such as the weakening effects of coffee, sugar, chocolate, cigarettes, alcohol, etc. Conversely, the strengthening effects of pure water and fresh fruit can convince people who are not educated in healthy eating that it's worth making changes in their diet.

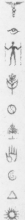

Probably the most useful self-help tool of all is the Emotional Stress Release technique, applied to present, past and future. Everyone, from the Managing Director to the worker on the factory floor, can benefit from this simple, powerful technique. Temporal tapping can be used to consolidate the changes that have been made. Not only do these techniques bring about improvements at the time; they can be used as ongoing self-help techniques at home as well as at work.

All these and other techniques can be taught in a single training session. They help to promote better working relationships, a positive attitude to work, and a sense of well-being not only at work but in life as a whole.

CORPORATE STRESS

A department in a large company was facing a substantial cut in budget resulting in some reorganization. Needless to say, this was causing the staff some stress and anxiety.

I was invited to run a training session for them. All the employees in the department attended the session, which combined Kinesiology and other management training skills.

During the training session they redefined their goals, as individuals and as a group. They saw the value of clear and positive communication, and learned self-help techniques to reduce stress, improve performance and creativity, and enhance their health through eating more wholesome foods.

Although some members had at first been unsure about the value of such a training, by the end of the session they were all pleased they had come, and felt they had benefited. They had created new ideas and plans for the future, and were feeling much more positive. They also felt much closer to each other, and were looking forward to better working relationships.

Christine Baldwin, the former occupational therapist mentioned earlier in this chapter, has for the last four years worked in private practice as a hypnotherapist. Since also becoming a qualified Kinesiologist, her work has undergone dramatic changes:

> I am more aware of the interaction between the mind and body. For instance, someone who comes to see me with a drink problem may have a chemical imbalance as well as emotional conflicts causing the alcohol dependence. The same applies to a smoker who finds it difficult to quit smoking, to a person with a weight problem, or a depressive, and so on. Almost every problem that clients present with for hypnotherapy needs Kinesiological investigation first.
>
> One of the most common physical causes of emotional problems, headaches, insomnia, etc., is Candidiasis (Candida Albicans). There may also be allergies causing a whole range of problems. Desensitizing clients to the allergen can improve both their mental and physical well-being.

Kinesiology also offers short-cuts to the therapist whose clients are resistant to hypnosis, perhaps through fear of what they may discover, or of losing control:

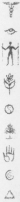

> I have often uncovered traumas using Kinesiological regression after coming against resistance. I am not suggesting that Kinesiology can take the place of hypnotherapy where there are deeply repressed incidents, but I have done useful work using the same NLP techniques that I use in hypnosis. I have always used Emotional Stress Release during hypnosis when there seemed to be no other way of relieving the stress of an inner conflict, and it works like a charm!

With some clients I switch from hypnosis to Kinesiology to counselling and back again, whatever I feel is the best way of resolving the client's problems. I used all the skills I have acquired where appropriate, including reflexology, Shiatsu, massage, dowsing, and so on.

Using hypnotherapy with Kinesiology, Christine has treated a wide variety of problems, including depression, eating problems; phobias, and anxieties generally. Some cases are quite simple – nerves before an exam or a driving test may be treatable in one or two sessions, for instance. More complicated cases involving childhood or other past traumas can take longer.

ANXIETY AND PHOBIAS

A professional man of 30 sought help for severe anxiety, nervous symptoms, relationship problems and low self-esteem. He had a number of fears, including fear of heights, of lifts, of being a passenger in a car, of snakes and of crocodiles. He also suffered from irritable bowel syndrome.

The practitioner knew that she would need to find the root cause of his emotional problems. Her Kinesiology assessment found that he had adrenal exhaustion, and numerous energy blocks in the meridian system. He told her he had feelings of being trapped and losing control, and an obsession with death that had started at the age of 11.

During the second to sixth sessions, hypnosis was used to regress him to childhood, using NLP techniques to ease his anxious memories. It emerged that he had witnessed a suicide as a child, which connected with his fears and phobias.

During the next three sessions Emotional Stress Release and other balancing techniques helped him to regress in memory without too much stress. The sessions continued with hypnoanalysis, and by the fifteenth session, using Kinesiology again, he'd been found to have a number of allergies, particularly to milk (which made him feel jittery), for which de-sensitization techniques were used.

He broke off treatment for two months, after which he returned for another four sessions. He was now able to hypnotize himself, and had a very vivid recall of past events, the effects of which were neutralized with NLP and Kinesiology techniques, as well as Bach Flower Remedies.

At this time his treatment is not yet complete, but he is much more relaxed, and more confident in personal relationships.

ENERGY MEDICINE

Kinesiology itself could be classified in the field of energy medicine, with its strong connection with the acupuncture system. It is also highly compatible with other forms of energy medicine, including healing.

ACUPUNCTURE

Marek Urbanowicz, MAc, MTAcS, is an acupuncturist trained in Kinesiology. As he points out, the primary difference between acupuncture and Kinesiology is that Kinesiology has grown out of a twentieth-century structural view of the body based on chiropractic, whereas acupuncture is one aspect of Traditional Oriental Medicine, going back thousands of years.

Kinesiology has taken certain basic models from oriental medicine including the meridians and the concept of *qi* energy. Within oriental medicine itself there are different schools of thought, and Kinesiology has adopted and used parts of what is known as the Five Elements model. As Kinesiology continues to expand, it may adopt other models of acupuncture. At this early stage in its

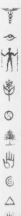

history, Kinesiology has a very simplistic approach to acupuncture theory. However, it has succeeded in de-mystifying some of the more esoteric ideas by demonstrating their validity via manual muscle testing.

The use of acupuncture alone only addresses one aspect of the Triad of Health, and does not treat directly the body's chemistry or structure. However, it is possible to effect changes in these areas indirectly. An acupuncturist who uses Kinesiology is able to view the patient from a much broader perspective. He or she can include structural factors, food sensitivities and nutritional needs, and can also view the patient from both a Western and an Oriental perspective. Consequently, a patient who visits a Kinesiologist/acupuncturist will have a broader and more thorough diagnosis, and will be more likely to benefit from treatment.

M.E./CHRONIC FATIGUE SYNDROME

Miss S., a student of 28, was suffering numerous symptoms related to M.E./Chronic Fatigue Syndrome, including chest infections and the eating disorder bulimia. She had had hepatitis and glandular fever in the past, and had a tendency to thrush, cystitis and Candidiasis. She had bad period pains, and mood swings. She had been treated medically with intravenous antibiotics and an investigatory laparoscopy.

A predominant imbalance was found in the lung and colon meridians (which relate to the Metal element). Using Kinesiology, Miss S. was found to be intolerant to wheat, corn, sugar, and rennet, and deficient in magnesium. She was also suffering from metal toxicity, with an overload of lead and aluminium in her system. Structurally, she had a tilted pelvis, TMJ problems, cranial faults and an ICV problem.

After being treated with Kinesiology there was an immediate improvement in several areas. The ICV correction brought about an instant reduction of her stomach bloating, diarrhoea, headaches and irritability.

After long-term treatment using both acupuncture and Kinesiology, there has been an 80 per cent improvement in the M.E. She now exercises regularly with no ill-effects, and has returned to her studies, working full-time as well as running a busy household. Her periods are improved, with only occasional discomfort. There has also been a reduction in the length and frequency of her chest infections. She can now tolerate corn in her diet on a regular basis, and occasionally, wheat. The thrush recurs very rarely, and the Candida is under control. She has not had bulimia for five years.

HEALING

Kinesiology is itself a form of natural healing, but in this section we are referring to healing as practised by healers who use a range of energy treatments such as laying on of hands, gems, colour, and sound, working with the body's subtle energy to bring about changes in the physical body.

Healing, also known as spiritual healing and etheric healing among other titles, has long been a source of mystery and superstition. The acceptance of the energy body and energy systems helps, at least in part, to explain why 'laying on of hands' by a sensitive therapist can actually produce physical changes in another person.

Kinesiology muscle testing provides a unique bridge between the physical body and the body's subtle energies. In Chapter 2 we referred to Dr Richard Gerber's description of the acupuncture system as the interface between the physical body and the subtle energy fields. When Kinesiology muscle tests are used to obtain an energy read-out of the meridians, they are also giving a read-out of the subtle energy fields.

The aura, the healers' word for the subtle energy field around the body, extends outwards and can be seen and felt (by sensitives) from as far away as one metre. Muscle testing can be used to find imbalances in the aura with great precision, pinpointing their location and distance from the body. These imbalances have an effect on the physical body: having found the exact location of the subtle energy imbalance the practitioner can either hold his or her hand in that area until the energy is balanced (this may be all that is needed), or find out which of a choice of energy treatments will be most effective in correcting it – including homoeopathic remedies, Bach Flower Remedies, essential oils, gems, crystals, colour or sound.

Kinesiology demystifies the realm of healing. Using the physical muscle test to identify imbalances in subtle energy which cannot normally be seen is a wonderful way of demonstrating the existence of this subtle energy, particularly to people who are unfamiliar with it. For some people, this is the first real proof that there is more to the physical body than meets the eye; it opens up a whole new and exciting awareness about themselves, and changes their beliefs.

It is not only clients whose minds are opened in this way. Many Touch For Health students discover their own sensitivity and healing potential for the first time while participating in a basic workshop. They start to feel the energy in the meridians, to tune in to the Emotional Stress Release points and allow the sensitivity of their fingers to find exactly which place to touch and how much pressure to use.

In other words, they discover that they have the sensitivity that previously they supposed only 'healers' possessed. We are all potential healers, and some people just need to discover this potential in themselves. Kinesiology provides a truly natural way to make this discovery.

I was teaching a group about Kinesiology and healing. One of the members had had a pre-menopausal problem of continuous menstrual bleeding over many months, resulting in anaemia. Neither hospital treatment nor hormone therapy had relieved her.

In the group exercise her partner discovered, through muscle testing, an imbalance in the woman's energy field about 18 in/45 cm from her body, over her uterus. The partner simply held her hand in the woman's energy field for a minute or two, removing it when it felt right to stop.

The next day the woman phoned me up, thrilled and delighted, to report that her bleeding had stopped. Regular balancing with friends from the group helped to maintain her improvement, and quickly restored her vitality.

BACH FLOWER REMEDIES

Bach Flower Remedies are often used by natural therapists and healers – and also by some medical doctors – to support patients in making emotional changes. These very pure remedies, made from plant essences and spring water, are aimed at transforming specific states of mind, and are believed to work via the subtle energy fields; there are 38 individual plant remedies, plus a Rescue Remedy which is a composite of five of these.

Charles Benham, an holistic therapist, uses Bach Flower Remedies among a range of holistic techniques in his own branch of Kinesiology, Optimum Health Balance.

AN ALLERGY TO CATS

A married woman of 32 came to see Charles Benham suffering from a severe allergic reaction to cat hair, which she had had for many years without responding to medical or natural

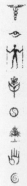

treatment. Within a few seconds of exposure her eyes and nose would become irritated, red and puffy, she had prolonged sneezing fits, and a fiery rash would cover her face and neck.

Assessment confirmed that, apart from this, her health was good. A vial containing cat hairs was placed on her navel, which immediately induced profound and general muscle weakness. With the vial in place, a variety of treatment modalities and remedies were tested.

The result was the selection of four Bach Flower Remedies – Heather, Impatiens, Mimulus and White Chestnut. Two drops of each were diluted in water, and the woman was instructed to take four drops of this mixture three times daily for nine days. The woman was given her first dose on the spot, which immediately cancelled the weak response to the cat hair sample.

Six weeks later she telephoned in great delight to say that her problem was over; the previous afternoon a friend's cat had settled on her lap, producing no adverse reactions. She had one slight recurrence, for which the same remedies were indicated, and was advised to get her own supply to take if the need arose. In fact it did not. Her allergy never recurred.

RELIEF FOR MIGRAINES

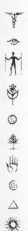

Another client was a married woman of 51. For ten years she had suffered about once a month with a severe migraine, including nausea, depression, and a feeling of coldness, lasting two or three days. Acupuncture and homoeopathy had failed to help. She also thought she was allergic to citrus fruits, and mentioned that she had suffered pain in her left hip and leg since a car accident several years earlier.

Testing revealed a definite link between the migraine and the allergic reaction, and the two in combination were therefore brought to the client's awareness. Additional testing revealed a pelvic displacement on the left side of the body, with 'active' scar tissue on the left leg resulting from the accident. (Active scar tissue can break up the energy flow in the related meridian.)

Through muscle testing the client's body selected as treatment the Bach Flower Remedies Clematis and Scleranthus. She was to take two drops of each in water four times daily for ten days. This was the only treatment required. On re-testing, all the problems previously revealed appeared to have been eliminated.

The client continues to attend at six-monthly intervals for 'maintenance' visits. Her migraine has never recurred. The woman's left leg, which had been badly injured, still gives her some trouble from time to time, but her regular visits keep this under control.

KINESIOLOGY FOR ANIMALS

Kinesiology techniques can be applied to animals just as to human beings, and among his other developments, Dr Harry Howell has made an in-depth study of this with Animal Kinesiology (AnK).

As he points out, some vets today are following the general trend towards using natural medicines, treating their patients with acupuncture and homoeopathy, and in some cases with chiropractic and healing. Legally only qualified vets are allowed to treat animals, but, as Harry Howell points out, the law does not prevent an owner from helping his or her own animal:

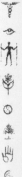

My approach has been to develop a system which can be taught to owners, using a surrogate to muscle test their animal.

All animals have the same organs as humans; only the locations are different. They also have acupuncture meridians. AnK works on much the same principle as Kinesiology, inasmuch as the therapist (or owner) challenges the various points on the animal's anatomy while, at the same time, testing the surrogate's muscle. The treatment is the same as for humans, except that I tend to use herbal tinctures in preference to tablets, as these are easier to administer.

MAJOR, THE CAT

Major, then aged two, had been suffering progressive loss of weight, increased thirst (accompanied by increased output of urine) and vomiting; his coat was becoming dry and coarse, with patches of eczema. He had been put on two successive courses of antibiotics, followed by a course of steroids. There had been no beneficial response, and the vet had told Major's owner that the cat's life expectancy was one to three months.

This was clearly a kidney problem, confirmed by using Kinesiology. Diagnosis was the easy part, however: it took a lot of eliminating of apparently appropriate remedies before discovering those that were actually needed. These were two homoeopathic remedies, *Arsenicum Album* and *Natrum Muriaticum*.

A change of diet was also recommended, particularly the elimination of dried food, which often causes kidney problems, especially in male cats.

Within four weeks Major's symptoms had completely disappeared. Two years later, at the time of writing, he is in prime health.

CONCLUSION

Any new discipline – and Kinesiology first appeared in the mid-1960s – takes time to spread and gain recognition. Those professionals who are using it are in no doubt about its reliability and effectiveness. It is to be hoped that many more will follow in their pioneering footsteps. Information about the application of Kinesiology in specialized fields can be obtained directly from specialists themselves, or from various training organizations. See Appendix B for a list of contacts.

CONCLUSION

We hope that this book has achieved its purpose: to introduce you to the world of Kinesiology and give you some idea of the scope of this rapidly developing and exciting new field.

Because Kinesiology has grown organically and is not associated with a single person or organization, it is not a clearly defined body of knowledge. We have attempted to pull together the many different aspects of this field, and to define some of the common areas. By writing about acceptable and unacceptable standards of muscle testing we also aim to educate the public about what to expect, and thus to reduce the number of people who use muscle testing inadequately, to the detriment of Kinesiology and their clients. We have deliberately excluded instructions for muscle testing, which should be learned under supervision from trained instructors.

Since the spread of Kinesiology world-wide took place via Touch For Health, which was designed for non-professional laypersons, its development has not been supervised by a professional governing body. Until recently ICAK was the only such body, and its criteria for membership exclude the majority of Kinesiologists practising world-wide. However, as a growing number of professional therapists and others adopt

Kinesiology and incorporate it into their work, or use it as a therapy in its own right, the need has emerged for standards and accreditation and most countries are now setting standards for professional practice.

In a book of this length it has not been possible to provide in-depth information on any one area. Many specialist books have been written focusing on particular systems and branches. Most of these require some basic training in Kinesiology before they can be fully appreciated.

It is our hope that the information given here will lead you to want to explore Kinesiology further. If you already enjoy good health, you may want to include Kinesiology as part of your fitness programme. If you have a health problem, you might consider consulting a Kinesiologist for treatment. If you are interested in self-help health enhancement, you might be interested in attending a Touch For Health workshop. If you are already studying Kinesiology, you may consider training in a particular branch. And if you are already a professional health practitioner, you may want to enhance your work by adding Kinesiology to your existing range of skills. If you work in other fields, such as management or education, you might also find it valuable to apply Kinesiology in your work. Whatever your background, there is scope for further training, develop-ment or participation.

Finally, we trust that you now have a greater appreciation of the interrelationship of your body, mind and spirit, and of how Kinesiology can be used to discover and enhance these connections. Kinesiology bridges the gap between the physical and non-physical planes, and enables you to experience directly for yourself, through muscle testing and energy balancing, the invisible and intangible aspects that play such a vital role in health and well-being.

APPENDIX A

TOUCH FOR HEALTH (TFH) LEVELS 1–4 AND FOUNDATION KINESIOLOGY PRACTITIONER (FKP) PARTS 1–2 SUMMARY OF WORKSHOP/COURSE CONTENT

Introduction to Kinesiology and Touch For Health

Postural awareness

Muscles and Muscle testing

Acupuncture meridians and subtle energy assessment

The muscle/meridian/organ/gland energetic connection

Communication and Goal-setting

Muscle biofeedback, indicator muscle testing and application

Pre-tests

Six standard corrections/treatments

Additional standard tests and corrections

Selecting and prioritizing corrections and treatment

Principles of balancing and balancing options

Introduction to acupuncture energy concepts

5 elements metaphor and correspondences: emotions, colours, sounds, etc.

Postural analysis, postural release and reactive muscles

Emotional stress release (ESR)

Pain control

Food sensitivity testing

Self-help

Note: All the above subjects are presented in the TFH work-shops and on FKP courses, though the order in which each subject is presented and the depth with which it is studied varies.

APPENDIX B

TRAINING CENTRES AND CONTACTS

When possible, please enclose a stamped addressed envelope with any enquiries.

INTERNATIONAL KINESIOLOGY ORGANIZATIONS

International College of Applied Kinesiology (ICAK) (UK), Metabolics, Eastcott House, Eastcott, Devizes, Wiltshire SN10 4PL. Tel. 01380 813139. Fax. 01380 813078.

International College of Applied Kinesiology (ICAK), 6405 Metcalf Avenue STE 503, Shawnee, Kansas 66202, USA. Tel. (913) 384–5336.

Three-in-One Concepts, 2001 West Magnolia Boulevard, Suite C, Burbank, California 91596–1704, USA. Tel. (818) 841–4786. Fax. (818) 841–0007.

Educational Kinesiology Foundation, P.O. Box 3396, Ventura, California 93006–3396, USA. Tel. (800) 356–2109. Fax. (805) 650–0524.

International Kinesiology College (ICK), Headquarters, Hurbigstrasse 157, CH-8454 Buchberg, Switzerland. Tel./Fax. 0041–1–867 14 77.

Touch For Health Foundation, 1174 North Lake Avenue, Pasadena, California 91104–3797, USA. Tel. (818) 794–1181.

International Association of Specialized Kinesiologists (I–ASK) (for worldwide information) I–ASK Home Office, P.O. Box 415, Bristol, Vermont, USA 05443–0415. Tel. (802) 453–6196. Fax. (802) 453–6197.

KINESIOLOGY ORGANIZATIONS (UK)

The Kinesiology Federation (for nationwide UK information) P.O. Box 7891, London SW19 1ZB. Tel. 0181–545 0255.

Association for Systematic Kinesiology (ASK) (for nationwide UK information), 39 Browns Road, Surbiton, Surrey KT5 8ST. Tel. 0181–399 3215.

Touch For Health Centre (for nationwide UK information) 30 Sudley Road, Bognor Regis, W. Sussex PO21 1ER. Tel. 01243 841689.

Touch For Health (England)
c/o Natalie Davenport, Garden Flat, 143 Iffley Road, Oxford OX4 1EJ. Tel. 01865 798885.

Middle England School of Kinesiology
81 Lancashire Street, Melton Road, Leicester LE4 7AF. Tel. 0116 266 1962.

Foundation Kinesiology Practitioner (FKP)
c/o Maggie la Tourelle, Integrated Practitioner Training (IPT), 70A Caversham Road, London NW5 2DS. Tel. 0171–485 4215.

PKP
c/o Gail McKerrow, 23 Maitland Avenue, Musselburgh EH21 6DZ. Tel./Fax. 0131–665 9577.

Educational Kinesiology, BioKinesiology, Hyperton-X
c/o Kay McCarroll, MC, MIPC, DHP, Body Balance UK Ltd., 12 Golders Rise, London NW4 2HR. Tel. 0181-202 9747. Fax. 0181-202 3890.

Three-in-One Concepts
c/o Daphne Clarke, 178 Elmer Road, Middleton-on-Sea, Sussex PO22 6JA. Tel./Fax. 01243 58335.

Health Kinesiology
c/o Jane Thurnell-Read, MSc, Grad. IPM, Sea View, Long Rock, Penzance, Cornwall, TR20 8JF. Tel. 01736 19030.

Clinical Kinesiology
c/o Ashley Robinson, DO, MRO, 5 High Street, Kington, Herefordshire, HR5 3AX.

KINESIOLOGY AND OTHER FIELDS: CONTACT PEOPLE, UK

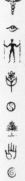

Acupuncture
Marek Urbanowicz, The Crescent Clinic of Complementary Medicine, 37 Vernon Terrace, Brighton, E. Sussex BN1 3JH. Tel. 01273 202221.

Bates Method (Eyesight Training)
Anthony Attenborough, 128 Merton Road, London SW18 5SP. Tel. 0181–874 7337.

Chiropractic
Richard Cook, DC, 82 Lowlands Road, Harrow, Middx. HA1
3AN. Tel. 0181–864 6768.

Counselling
Maggie la Tourelle, 70A Caversham Road, London NW5 2DS.
Tel. 0171–485 4215.

Dentistry
Mr R. J. A. Sudworth, BDS, LDS, RCS (Eng.), 132 Queens Road,
Clifton, Bristol BS8 1LQ. Tel. 0117 973 4737.

Education
Daphne Clarke, 178 Elmer Road, Middleton-on-Sea, Sussex,
PO22 6JA. Tel./Fax. 01243 58335.

Healing
Maggie la Tourelle, 70A Caversham Road, London NW5 2DS.
Tel. 0171–485 4215.

Hypnotherapy
Ms Christine Baldwin, SROT, MBAOT, DipCOT, MWFH,
The Foxgrove Clinic, Borers Arms Road, Copthorne, Crawley,
W. Sussex RH10 3LH. Tel. 01342 716505.

Medical Herbalism
Daphne Benjamin, MNIMH, Tonbridge Natural Therapy
Centre, Barton House, 11 London Road, Tonbridge, Kent TN10
3AB. Tel. 01732 355868.

Nutritional Therapy
Christine Baldwin, The Foxgrove Clinic, Borers Arms Road,
Copthorne, Crawley, W. Sussex RH10 3LH. Tel. 01342 716505.

Optimum Health Balance

Charles Benham, The Optimum Health Balance Centre, 15 Pinions Road, High Wycombe, Bucks. HP13 7AT.

Osteopathy

Christopher R. A. Smith, DO, MRO, Devizes, Wilts and Andover, Hants. Tel. 01380 813139 and 01264 323901.

TOUCH FOR HEALTH/KINESIOLOGY CONTACTS (OVERSEAS)

Toni Gralton, P.O. Box 164, Buderim, QLD 4556, Australia. Tel. 61–74–45 49 29. Fax. 61–74–45 33 19.

Gabriele Lehner, Akademie für AK, A–8362 Krauterdorf Sochau, Austria. Tel. 43–3387–3210. Fax. 43–3387–3212.

Dominique Monette, MD, 46 Ave. Ducpetiaux, B–1060 Brussels, Belgium. Tel./Fax. 32–2–537 64 61.

Clovis Horta Corréa, Rua Cupertino Durão 105/202, Leblon-Rio de Janeiro R/J, CEP 22441–030 Brazil. Tel. 55 21 259 7266. Fax. 55 21 240 4668.

Gerardo Vale, SQS 302 Bloco F, Apt. 202, Brasilia/DF 780 338 010, Brazil. Tel. 55 61 226 7889. Fax. 55 61 242 3669.

Michael De Lory, 2116 West, 8th Avenue, Vancouver, B.C., V6K 2A4, Canada. Tel. 1–604–737 77 79.

Grethe Fremming & Rolf Hausboel, Gardes Allé 8, DK–2900 Hellerup, Denmark. Tel. 45–31–62–45 30. Fax. 45–31–62 47 10.

Alfred Schatz & Susanne Degendorfer, Zasiusstrasse 67, D–79102 Freiburg, Germany. Tel. 49–761–7 33 08. Fax. 49–761–70 63 84.

Risteard De Barra, 84 Cappaghmore Clondalkin, Dublin 22, Ireland. Tel./Fax. 353–1–457 11 83.

Maurizio Piva, Via F. 11i Bianchi 5, I–25080 Maderno S/G BS, Italy. Tel./Fax. 39–365–64 15 53.

Aria den Hartog, Rijksweg 14–m, NL–6267 AG Cadier en Keer, Netherlands. Tel./Fax. 00–31–407–30–44.

Dr Bruce and Joan Dewe, P.O. Box 25–162, St Heliers, Auckland 1130, New Zealand. Tel. 64–9–575–2818. Fax. 64–9–575 2813.

Tom Arnold Pedersen, Herman Gransveil 7A, N–5034 Laksevag, Norway. Tel./Fax. 47–553–46 480.

Fernando Muñez Caravaca, ctra. de churra 6, E–30110 Murcia, Spain. Tel. 34–6883–4365. Fax. 34–6862–6711.

Institut für Kinesiologie, c/o Rosmarie & Bernhard Sonderegger Studer, Hurbigstrasse 157, CH–8454 Buchberg, Switzerland. Tel. 41–1–272 45 15. Fax. 41–1–867 14 77.

Jean-François Jaccard, 6 ch de la Fontaine, CH-1224 Chène-Bougeries, Switzerland. Tel./Fax. 41–22–349–56 00.

Dr John & Carrie Thie, 6162 La Gloria Drive, Malibu, California 90265, USA. Tel. 1–310–589 52 69. Fax. 1–310–589 53 69.

Arlene Green, 1717 Wildcat Creek Road, Chapel Hill, North Carolina, 27516, USA. Tel. 1–919–933 92 99.
Fax. 1–919–968 98 00.

Marguerite Murray, N.81 W.15062 Appleton Avenue, Menomonee Falls, Wisconsin 53051, USA. Tel. 1–414–253 49 05.
Fax. 1–414–253 49 05

BIBLIOGRAPHY AND FURTHER READING

These books can be found in specialist bookshops and some libraries. Entries asterisked (*) are American publications which can be purchased in Britain from Booklist, 78 Castlewood Drive, Eltham, London SE9 1NG. Tel./Fax. 0181–856 7717.

Elizabeth Andrews, *Muscle Management*, Thorsons, 1991.

Brian Butler, BA, *An Introduction to Kinesiology*, TASK, 1990.

*Roger Callahan, Ph.D., *How Executives Overcome the Fear of Public Speaking and Other Phobias* (previously *The Five Minute Phobia Cure*), Wilmington, DE: Enterprise Publishing Inc., 1985.

Leon Chaitow, *Candida Albicans: Could Yeast Be Your Problem?*, Thorsons, 1991.

Dianne M. Connelly, Ph.D., *Traditional Acupuncture: The Law of Five Elements*, Columbia, MD: The Center for Traditional Acupuncture Inc., 1979.

Anthea Courtenay, *Chiropractic for Everyone: Your Spine and Your Health*, Penguin Books, 1987.

Dr Stephen Davies and Dr Alan Stuart, *Nutritional Medicine*, Pan Books, 1987.

Dr Sheldon C. Deal, *New Life through Nutrition*, Tuscon: AZ: New Life Publishing, 1974.

182 *Paul E. Dennison, Ph.D. and Gail E. Dennison, *Edu-K for Kids*, Glendale, CA: Edu-Kinesthetics Inc., 1987.

*——, *Brain Gym*, Glendale, CA: Edu-Kinesthetics Inc., 1986.

*——, *Switching On*, Glendale, CA: Edu-Kinesthetics Inc., 1981.

Dr Bruce A. J. Dewe MD and Joan R. Dewe MA, *Professional Health Provider 1*, Auckland, NZ: Professional Health Practice Workshops, 1990.

Dr John Diamond MD, *Life Energy*, New York: Dodd, Mead & Co., 1985.

Dr Richard Gerber, MD, *Vibrational Medicine: New Choices for Healing Ourselves*, Santa Fe, NM: Bear & Co., 1988.

Gill Jacobs, *Candida Albicans: Yeast and Your Health*, Optima, 1990.

Ted J. Kaptchuk, *Chinese Medicine: The Web that Has No Weaver*, Rider & Co., 1983.

Joseph O'Connor and Ian McDermott, *Principles of NLP*, Thorsons, 1996.

*Jimmy Scott, Ph.D., *Cure Your Own Allergies in Minutes*, San Francisco: Health Kinesiology Publications, 1988.

*Gordon Stokes and Mary Marks DC, *Dr Sheldon Deal's Basic AK Workshop Manual*, Pasadena, CA: Touch For Health Foundation, 1983.

John F. Thie, DC, *Touch For Health Book*, Marina del Rey, CA: De Vorss & Co., 1973.

*Wayne Topping, Ph.D., *Success Over Distress*, Bellingham, WA: Topping International Institute, 1990.

*——, *Stress Release*, Bellingham, WA: Topping International Institute, 1991.

Tom and Carole Valentine, *Applied Kinesiology*, Thorsons, 1985.

David S. Walther DC, *Applied Kinesiology*, vols. 1 and 2, Pueblo, CO: Systems DC, 1981.

INDEX

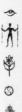

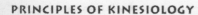

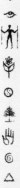